Insomnia Relief

How to Use Natural Sleep Aids to Get to Sleep and Stay Asleep

Deborah Bleecker, L.Ac., M.S.O.M.

Insomnia Relief

Deborah Bleecker, L.Ac., M.S.O.M.

Published by: Draycott Publishing

1st Edition

Printed in the United States of America

Draycott Publishing, LLC, Dallas, Texas

ISBN 978-1-940146-00-3

Library of Congress Control Number: 20-13949508

Disclaimer

This book is designed to provide information about the subject matter covered. It is sold with the understanding that the publisher and authors are not engaged in rendering legal, accounting, or other professional services. If medical or other expert assistance is required, the services of a competent professional should be sought.

Every effort has been made to make this book as complete and as accurate as possible. However, there may be mistakes both typographical and in content. Therefore, this text should be used only as a general guide and not as the ultimate source of information.

The purpose of this manual is to educate and entertain. The authors and Draycott Publishing, LLC shall have neither liability nor responsibility to any person or entity with respect to any loss or damage caused or alleged to be caused directly or indirectly by the information contained in this book.

If you do not wish to be bound by the above, you may return this book to the publisher for a full refund.

Acknowledgments

My thanks to my dad, you have stuck by me on my journey through life. You were there every step of the way in acupuncture school. I could not have done it without you.

I thank my mom, my first and number one patient. You dove into Chinese medicine and never doubted it for a minute. You've always been there as a support.

I would like to thank my teachers, Doctors Wang, He, and Wu. Your sacrifices have helped many people. You have helped not only all your students, but everyone they have helped also.

Thank you to the patients who encouraged me to write a book. I appreciate you and continue to learn from you.

I'm grateful to my editor Kathy Gaudry.

Dedication

This book is dedicated to acupuncturists everywhere. You work hard to learn your craft and struggle to make it when you get out of school. You persevere because you are determined to help people recover their health.

It is my hope that through my books, more people will understand how acupuncture works and will turn to you for help.

Table of Contents

Acupuncture and Chinese Medicine

Chapter 1

Is Insomnia Curable?

For every ailment, there is a root cause. If you treat the underlying cause of the ailment, it will be resolved. It might take some time to determine the cause of your insomnia, but once you start getting the care you need and take the necessary supplements, there is no reason to continue to suffer from insomnia.

What is normal?

It is important to sleep 7-8 hours per night. You can get slightly less or more than that, depending on your constitution, but 8 hours a night is a healthy goal. Many people sleep 6 hours a night for a long time and do not know the damage they are doing to their bodies. Your body does most of its healing and repair at night. If you do not get adequate sleep, your body cannot recover from daily stress and make the adequate hormones you need to be healthy.

As an acupuncturist, I have successfully treated insomnia with acupuncture and supplements for years. It is not common knowledge that acupuncture and Chinese herbs can treat insomnia. Most people have no idea acupuncture can help them with their sleep issues. Acupuncture and Chinese herbs can be used to treat your sleep at the same time we treat your other ailments. Acupuncture is effective because it treats the underlying imbalances that cause sleep problems. All acupuncturists are sleep and pain specialists. We treat them all day.

Although it is best if you can get acupuncture, I want you to be able to help yourself. I will give you tips on how to use supplements and acupressure to treat yourself.

As with any natural remedy, you need to give things time to work. We are treating the underlying cause of your insomnia. The goal is to help you get to sleep and stay asleep, without the need to take supplements or treatments of any kind.

While treating your insomnia, fatigue, anxiety, and stress will be reduced. This is a holistic treatment plan. In order to have healthy sleep, you have to treat the whole person. This is not just about taking sedative herbs. Our goal is complete health and good sleep.

Chapter 2

Adrenal Fatigue – Do You Feel Exhausted?

If you are under chronic stress, you can actually wear out your adrenal glands. When your body is under stress, the adrenals pump out excess adrenaline to cope with it. If you have high stress regularly, your adrenals can be depleted. They can lose the ability to excrete enough adrenaline for you to function normally. When this happens, you feel exhausted and rest does not improve how you feel.

Adrenal fatigue is a common cause of insomnia. You feel tired but wired. You just cannot shut down. I also believe this is a very common cause of depression. Unfortunately, few people are aware of this.

Adrenal fatigue is an epidemic right now. Our bodies were not designed to handle the constant stress we experience. Many people think they have anxiety, when in fact, their symptoms are caused by adrenal fatigue. If the adrenal glands are not supported with adequate vitamins and herbs, they will continue to decline until you break down. You do have a limit to the amount of stress your body can cope with. Anxiety is not in your head. There is always a physical cause.

Some common symptoms of adrenal fatigue are:

- Ability to handle stress is reduced. You become upset a lot more easily than usual.
- You do not think as clearly as you used to.
- You become confused easily and forget things.
- Muscle weakness
- Feelings of hopelessness and despair
- Exhausted feeling, sleep does not relieve fatigue
- Poor memory
- Decreased ability to deal with stress
- Trouble waking up in the morning, even after a full night's sleep
- Depression
- Insomnia
- Lightheadedness if you get up suddenly
- Dark circles under your eyes
- Decreased sex drive
- Unexplained headaches
- Low blood pressure
- Feel colder than usual
- Use caffeine and other stimulants to keep you going

Acupuncture and Chinese herbs are very effective to treat fatigue. In most cases, this will be enough to dramatically improve energy levels. However, if you have adrenal fatigue, you will need more time to recover and you will have to take vitamins and other supplements to restore your adrenals.

If you suspect you have adrenal fatigue, or even if you just feel tired, you can add some vitamins to your daily regimen that can improve your energy and overall health. If you are under stress and want to prevent the damage stress causes, adrenal supplements are very helpful.

The best book about adrenal fatigue is *Adrenal Fatigue, The 21st Century Stress Syndrome* by Dr. James Wilson. His site is www.adrenalfatigue.org. This book includes include lengthy questionnaires that will help you determine the status of your adrenals.

Adrenal fatigue is similar to a nervous breakdown. If your adrenals are weak enough, you cannot cope. You have no energy, can't sleep and everything irritates you more than usual. You feel on edge, anxious and overwhelmed.

Most people have never heard of adrenal fatigue. You can fully recover if you combine herbs with vitamins and a reduction in stress. Our modern stress levels are beyond what our bodies were designed to handle. If you are under a lot of stress, it is a good idea to be sure you take good quality vitamins to help your body cope.

Adrenal Fatigue Supplement Regimen

Vitamin C

Vitamin C - take at least 1,000 mg per day. When recovering from adrenal fatigue, you can take 8,000 mg per day minimum. The more vitamin C you take, the faster your adrenals recover. Much higher doses will just be excreted by the body if not needed. Vitamin C is specific to your adrenal glands. It also helps detox and boosts your immune system. If you take too much, you will have loose stools. If you are very deficient, you will be able to take very large amounts before it affects you. Bowel tolerance is when your body has enough vitamin C and any extra you take causes loose stools.

Vitamin C Supplements

Vitamin C, Vitamin Code by Garden of Life

Hy-Bio, Citrus Bioflavonoids Vitamins C, Rutin and Rose Hips by Solgar

Vitamin C – Citrus Bioflavonoids by Jarrow

B Vitamins

B vitamins are the stress and energy vitamins. They are quickly depleted when you are under stress. They are water soluble, so they just wash out of your body if you take more than you need. I found the Garden of Life Raw B vitamins to be the best brand. The line is called "Vitamin Code." These vitamins are fermented and enzyme-processed and absorbed far better than any brand I have tried.

Many vitamins are not absorbed well, even if they are high quality. When choosing supplements, a small dose of a higher quality and well absorbed vitamin is better than a large dose of a lower quality brand.

Siberian Ginseng

Siberian ginseng is a good energy tonic. It is an adaptogen, which means it helps your body adapt to and recover from stress. It can be taken long term. Even if you just take one capsule of the extract daily, it will improve your resistance to adrenal issues. Nature's Way and Solaray brands are my first choice.

Licorice Root

Helps replace adrenal hormones while your adrenals recover. Solaray and Nature's Way are good choices for herbs.

Cordyceps Sinensis

Cordyceps is used to improve kidney energy. It is a very strong energy tonic and can be taken long term. I like the Planetary Herbals brand and Nature's Way brand. This is one of the best energy tonic herbs you can take. It makes your lungs, heart, and kidneys stronger. Cordyceps is used for endurance, fatigue, and incontinence.

Fo-Ti (He Shou Wu)

He shou wu (fo-ti)– this herb is not listed in most supplement lists for adrenal fatigue, because it is not well-known in the West. It is used in Chinese medicine to strengthen the kidneys. It also improves hair growth and reduces grey hair. It is one of the best kidney tonics you can take. It is an "essence" tonic. It is also used for longevity.

The way you know it is improving hair growth is that you can easily see the difference at your hairline when you take it regularly. Within a month, you can see new hairs growing in. No, it will not increase arm hair or facial hair in women. It improves normal, healthy head hair growth. It will not give women hairy hands.

Fo-ti (he shou wu or polygonum multiflorum) is also used for infertility in men and women. The legend of this herb in Chinese medicine is that a man called "He" had premature grey hair and it grew in black again by using this herb. Golden Flower is a good brand. It is sold only through acupuncturists. Another good option is Sun Ten "Tang-kuei shou wu pills". This is a high quality extract of Dang gui, he shou wu, and Siberian ginseng. The He shou wu will improve hair growth, Dang gui will help regulate hormones and the Siberian ginseng is good for the adrenal glands. Sun Ten makes high quality extracts of Chinese herbs that are available online.

There are many supplements that are sold as hair tonics. The active ingredient is the fo-ti. They also often include biotin and other vitamins, but fo-ti is the most active ingredient. I regularly give this to my patients to improve hair growth. It is one of the most important longevity tonics in Chinese medicine.

Chapter 3

Calcium and Magnesium Deficiency

It is estimated that 80% of Americans have a deficiency in magnesium. Your body needs magnesium to relax your muscles. It uses calcium to contract muscles. Many people take calcium supplements alone as a single supplement. This is one of the worst things you can do.

Your body needs magnesium in order to absorb calcium. If you do not have enough magnesium, the calcium can just float around in your body and deposit in joints and other parts of your body. If you take magnesium by itself, that is not a problem. In fact, if you are magnesium deficient, you will want to take magnesium for a few months to replenish your blood levels.

It is estimated that 95% of women are deficient in calcium. The problem is that it is hard to absorb calcium from dairy products. Many calcium supplements are also not absorbed very well. It is more effective to take a supplement that contains calcium, magnesium, vitamin D, and other co-factors needed for absorption.

Symptoms of a calcium deficiency include:

- Muscle cramps
- Weak or brittle nails
- Fatigue
- Insomnia
- Brain fog
- Mood irregularities

Symptoms of a magnesium deficiency include:

- Stress
- Fatigue
- Inability to sleep
- Muscle tension, spasms, and cramps
- Anxiousness and nervousness
- Irritability
- Headaches
- Weakness
- PMS and hormonal imbalances
- Weakening bones
- Abnormal heart rhythm

Soft Drinks Deplete Mineral Levels

Soft drinks that have phosphoric acid in them are a common cause of calcium/magnesium deficiency. Your body has to buffer this acid to prevent damage to your tissues. It does this by pulling minerals from your blood first, if there is not enough to buffer the acid, it pulls minerals from the bones, your mineral storage depots. It needs calcium, magnesium, and other minerals to buffer the acid. If you drink a lot of soft drinks, you can easily deplete your minerals. If you have ever drunk soft drinks regularly, it is a good idea to replenish your calcium and magnesium levels. I am not telling you that you need to stop drinking all soft drinks, I just want you to be aware of your calcium/magnesium balance and take extra supplements to protect yourself.

I believe that our high soft drink consumption is contributing to the increase in osteoporosis and osteopenia. You can still recover from this by taking supplements that include calcium and magnesium.

Migraine Headaches

Magnesium deficiency is a common contributing factor in migraine headaches. Migraine headaches are basically tight muscles in the neck and shoulders that put pressure on the blood vessels and nerves leading to the brain. When you cut off normal blood flow, you will have pain. Acupuncture can help to relax the muscles and open up circulation to relieve migraines.

Not all migraines are caused by tight neck muscles. They can also be caused by blockage of normal blood flow in any area of your head and shoulders. In addition, a blockage of any meridian in the body can cause migraines and headaches. Sinus headaches can also initiate migraines.

In order to absorb calcium, you need magnesium, vitamin D, and other co-factors. If you take calcium supplements without magnesium, it is not absorbed well and can cause health issues such as deposition of calcium in places that you do not want calcium. If your body cannot absorb it, it is believed it can be deposited in your arteries. Calcium supplements should not be taken alone as a single mineral.

Calcium/Magnesium Supplements

Raw Calcium by Garden of Life

This product has been proven in many research studies to improve bone health. It is organic and is made from a marine algae called Algas calcareas. The trademarked name is Algae Cal. It includes 73 bone-building minerals and trace elements. Ingredients include Vitamin D, vitamin K, calcium, and magnesium. Since it is a whole food, it is absorbed better than other calcium/magnesium supplements.

Natural Calm Magnesium Drink

If you do not want to take magnesium tablets, you can take ionic magnesium powder. Natural Calm magnesium by Natural Vitality is an ionic magnesium powder that you mix with juice or water. It has 325 mg magnesium per 2 teaspoon serving. This is the minimum RDA for magnesium. If you are deficient, you might need to take a higher dose to replenish your body.

They also have a product called Natural Calm plus Calcium. It has per 3 teaspoon dosage: Vitamin C – 265 mg, Vitamin D – 105 IU, Calcium gluconate – 210 mg, Magnesium citrate – 320 mg, Potassium – 105 mg, Boron – 265 mcg.

There are other brands of powdered magnesium. The problem is that they include B vitamins. You don't want to take your magnesium supplement in the evening if it includes B vitamins. Taking B vitamins will boost your energy, just as you are trying to calm down.

Magnesium Glycinate

Chelated magnesium Glycinate is the best absorbed magnesium supplement. The chelated type of minerals is better absorbed. Chelation is when the mineral is bound to an amino acid, so your body will allow more through the intestinal wall. Your body protects you from absorbing large amounts of minerals at one time.

It does this by causing a flushing of your intestines when you take too much. The Solgar brand of "Chelated Magnesium" is very well absorbed.

Chapter 4

Menopause and Hormonal Imbalances

It Starts at Age 35

If you are a woman, you need to know that changes in your hormones will occur long before you start getting hot flashes. Your ovaries reduce production of estrogen and progesterone. You can start having odd symptoms and not be aware that they are caused by a decline in your hormone levels.

Your hormone levels can start to decline in your late thirties and early forties. The reason I am including this information here is that hormone deficiencies are a common cause of insomnia.

Taking herbal sedatives like Valerian root will unlikely be enough to cure your insomnia, if you have a hormone deficiency. You might need to take supplements to improve hormone levels. Acupuncture and Chinese herbs are also effective to balance your hormone levels.

Perimenopause

Perimenopause is a time of transition when a woman's ovaries start to reduce the production of hormones.

This period of hormone reduction that starts in your thirties.

Common symptoms of perimenopause are:

- Irregular periods
- Vaginal dryness
- Mood swings
- Reduced libido
- Insomnia
- Hot flashes
- Night sweats

At this stage of menopause, your hormone production is declining and your body is trying to make the adjustments it needs to stay in balance.

As time goes on, your hormone levels continue to decline. This is a natural part of the aging process. That does not mean you have to continue to suffer the symptoms of a hormone deficiency. At the perimenopause stage, addressing hormone issues does not take as long as treating it once you become menopausal.

Adrenal Fatigue

When your ovaries reduce the amount of hormones they make, your adrenal glands are supposed to increase hormone production. If you have adrenal fatigue, it is very hard for your adrenals to make sufficient hormones.

The severity of your symptoms is determined by how hormone deficient you are. About 80% of women will suffer from hot flashes and night sweats. If you have never had this, you will not have any idea of how bad it is. It is like being on fire internally. It does not feel like the room is hot. It feels like you are on fire. Men can get hot flashes also; they suffer from the same hormone decline as women. They suffer more from a decline of testosterone.

Testosterone

All of your hormones decline as you age. Your testosterone, progesterone, and estrogen production is reduced. Testosterone is usually associated with libido in men, and it does the same thing in women. It is very easy to recover normal testosterone levels with herbs. Herbs like Cordyceps replenish your kidney energy, which improves the ability of your body to make its own hormones. It can often be taken long term.

Horny Goat Weed

Taking kidney tonics like Horny goat weed as a single herb is not recommended for anyone. This is a Chinese herb, but it is not used alone as a single herb. In Chinese medicine, it is used in small amounts, less than 10% and is used for less than a month in most cases.

This herb should not be taken without a prescription from a licensed acupuncturist. It is called "yin yang huo" and it is very warm energetically. It is not appropriate for most people, even when combined with other herbs in a formula. If you are taking this herb for energy levels or libido, please see the andropause for information on this. You can easily cause a hormone imbalance that causes insomnia by taking this herb. Hormones are about balance. Since all your hormones decline, it is best to treat them together.

Best Libido Tonics

In lieu of taking herbs like horny goat weed, I want you to know the healthy libido tonics. The best libido tonics can be taken long term and will only build up your energy without causing negative side effects. The best libido tonics are Goji berries, American ginseng, and Cordyceps.

As an herbalist, I am frustrated with herbs like horny goat weed being sold as a single herb and having unsuspecting people taking it and not knowing their symptoms come from taking the herb. If you take this herb for longer than you need it, you can quickly develop an excess of testosterone.

Symptoms of too much testosterone:

- Hot flashes
- Irritability
- Insomnia
- Dark facial hair in women

All these are symptoms of too much testosterone, relative to estrogen and progesterone. Even if you need testosterone, it is best to take an herbal tonic like Cordyceps that can be taken long term. It is a gentler tonic and it strengthens your kidneys to help them improve your hormone levels, not just the testosterone. Your acupuncturist can help you choose the best tonic for your situation.

Dark Facial Hair in Women

If you have already taken too much horny goat weed or just have dark facial hair due to an estrogen deficiency or other hormonal imbalance, this can be addressed with either the phytoestrogen formulas or taking American ginseng long term. American ginseng is a good tonic for people over 50. It is considered superior to Panax ginseng for those over 50. It helps to restore what your body loses as you age.

The most common age for menopause to occur is 50. Symptoms of hormonal deficiency can start in your late thirties. One of the most common and well-known symptoms of perimenopause and menopause is hot flashes.

Most common symptoms of menopause:

- Hot flashes
- Night sweats
- Irregular periods
- Vaginal dryness
- Mood swings
- Loss of libido

Other possible symptoms:

- Fatigue
- Hair loss or thinning
- Insomnia
- Memory lapses
- Bloating
- Brittle nails
- Irregular heartbeat
- Panic and anxiety
- Depression
- Breast pain
- Joint pain
- Muscle tension
- Dry, itchy skin
- Loss of skin elasticity
- Reduction of eyelashes
- Difficulty concentrating
- Dizziness
- Incontinence
- Bloating
- Anxiety

- Depression
- Irritability
- Headaches
- Electric shock sensation
- Gum problems
- Digestive problems
- Osteoporosis

There are many options to treat the symptoms of perimenopause and menopause.

Natural Remedies for Hot Flashes

If you suffer from hot flashes, herbal remedies can often treat them quickly. There are many herbs that balance your hormones. Some of the herbs are believed to contain estrogen like compounds and some just stimulate your body to make its own hormones. Once you already have hot flashes, the herbs that stimulate your body to make hormones might not be fast-acting enough for you. You might want to relieve the symptoms as quickly as possible.

The fastest way to relieve hot flashes and improve sleep is to take supplements that improve your hormone levels.

Solaray PhytoEstrogen is a good supplement for menopausal symptoms. One of my patients started having hot flashes and took 4 pills 3 times in one day and completely stopped getting hot flashes in 24 hours. It also quickly improves sleep and calms you down. You will need to experiment with your dosage to determine what is right for you. Your hormonal needs will also change over time.

Solaray PhytoEstrogen Ingredients:

Per 4 capsules:

Non GMO Soy (Glycine Max) (Bean Extract) 2 grams- Isoflavones

Mexiyam – Dioscorea Composita -200 mg

Black Cohosh – Cimicifuga Racemosa- 40 mg

Dong Quai- Angelica Sinensis – 40 mg

Other ingredients: Ginger root, licorice root, saw palmetto berry, and pygeum bark extract. Per Solaray, these ingredients were not considered active ingredients and they did not disclose amounts.

The dosage is 4 per day.

Solaray PhytoEstrogen Plus EFA's

Solaray also has a product with essential fatty acids in it, called Solaray PhytoEstrogen EFA. I personally do not like to combine herbs with any type of oil. Once the oil goes rancid, it will ruin the herbs. Oils should be stored in the refrigerator when possible. This product has Borage oil, Flax oil and evening primrose oil. These oils help your body with hormone balance. Taking these oils is good, but it is not my preference to combine oils with herbs in the same capsule. The likelihood of it going rancid is too high. Solaray is one of my favorite herb companies, but I believe the oil should be taken in a separate supplement.

Supplement manufacturers also sometimes include fish oil in supplements like glucosamine. Fish oil is good for your joints, because it is a natural anti-inflammatory and has many health benefits. But, fish oil should be refrigerated also. Nordic Naturals is a good choice for fish oil and it is not combined in other supplements.

There are many other supplements for menopausal symptoms. They each have different ingredients and different claims. You might have good results with one product and not with another one that is similar.

Over The Counter Supplements for Hormone Isssues

Remifemin

Black Cohosh extract- 20 mg per tablet.

Promensil

Red clover extract- 220 mg of red clover extract and 40 mg of isoflavones.

Your success with different supplements will be determined by how low your estrogen levels are and your body's chemistry. Everyone is different.

Hot Flash by Source Naturals also is a good combination formula.

Hot Flash by Source Naturals Ingredients:

Per 3 tablets:

2.1 grams Genistein rich soy extract, yielding 63 mg Isoflavones

Black Cohosh Extract – 160 mg

Dong Quai-150 mg

Licorice root extract- 150 mg

Chaste tree berry extract (Vitex)- 100 mg

Taking herbs in combination is stronger than taking a single herb. You get the benefits of all the herbs in the formula. Vitex (Chase tree berry) has been used for centuries to balance female hormone levels.

Herbs Used for Menopause Include:

Wild Yam, also called Mexican Yam – Dioscorea Villosa

- Estrogenic
- Anti-inflammatory
- Relieves muscle spasms, cramping pain
- Tight muscles

Black Cohosh – Cimicifuga Racemosa

- Native American remedy
- Relieves spasm
- Mild sedative/nervine

- Does not appear to contain estrogen, it can take 2-3 weeks to see if it will be effective for you.

Red Clover —Trifolium Pratense- Blood purifier, Blood thinner, Isoflavones

Black Cohosh Extract from Planetary Herbals

Black Cohosh root extract 160 mg, Calcium 109 mg

Soybean extract

The Asian diet contains up to 20 times the amount of phytoestrogens of the typical diet in the West. This might explain why fewer women in Asia have menopausal symptoms like hot flashes. Soybeans contain phytosterols and isoflavones that have been shown to bind to the same receptor sites as estrogen. Soybean extract is in the supplements PhytoEstrogen from Solaray and Hot Flash by Source Naturals.

Synthetic Estrogen

It is now well known that taking synthetically derived estrogen could increase your risk of cancer and other illnesses. When you chemically isolate something and make it into a drug, it is more likely to cause side effects.

In order to make a pharmaceutical drug for hormone deficiencies, drug companies must be able to patent it. In order to patent it, they have to isolate components of the herb. They cannot patent an herb, so they must try to isolate what they believe is the active ingredient.

Herbal remedies have many different components in them. One herbal component will reduce the bad side effects of another component. That is why herbs are often better tolerated. The dozens or hundreds of active ingredients balance each other out.

This is how Chinese herbal remedies are made. An herb that is toxic or too strong if taken alone is combined with other herbs to treat illnesses. It is about the balance. If you take an herb and say that you have found THE ingredient that is "active," you have just made a drug. You have isolated a compound and removed the other compounds that were balancing it.

Standardized herbs are different. These herbs are often extracted and tested to be sure they contain enough of the compound believed to be most effective. It is a quality assurance issue, not isolating one ingredient and selling that as a single remedy. The best herb companies test the potency of their herbs.

If you have symptoms, it is because there is something out of balance or missing in your body. These remedies have been used for centuries to address hormonal issues.

You should consult with your physician if you are concerned. If you are on medications, you should always consult with the prescribing doctor about supplements. Most herbs reduce the viscosity of blood. They make blood flow better, by making it less sticky. This is especially contraindicated for people on blood thinning drugs.

In addition to supplements in pill form, there are also topical creams and sprays with progesterone and estrogen in them.

Progesterone Cream: Source Naturals, Smoky Mountain Naturals

Estrogen Cream: Smoky Mountain Naturals - Natural Estrogen/Estriol Cream (Bioidentical), Source Naturals Phyto-estrogen cream

If you take progesterone or estrogen products, you might notice they can make you feel sleepy and relaxed. You might not notice it the first time you take it, but over time you could. Taking these products in the evening could reduce the side effects. Of course, if you have insomnia, you like feeling sleepy. Addressing hormonal imbalances that are causing your insomnia is important. It will take a little time for you to find what balance is right for you.

Each of these products has dosage information that should be followed as they all have different ingredients and strengths. It is very easy to use too much of the hormone creams. The dose is ¼ teaspoon. Your dosage should be according to your needs.

I am not giving medical advice about any of these supplements. Please consult your medical doctor or other healthcare practitioner for advice.

Sleepiness

You might notice that you feel a little drowsy if you take a lot of phytoestrogen pills at one time. It is not the kind of sleepiness you get from medications. It is just a calm and relaxed feeling that you probably have not felt for a long time if you are hormone deficient.

It will take some time to determine how many pills you need to take to balance out your hormone levels. The dosage on the bottle might not be enough for you. Your dosage over time might change also. If you have adrenal fatigue and live a high stress life, you might need a little higher dosage than someone who does not.

The natural flow of hormone production is to make a little more testosterone (yang) in the morning and more yin (estrogen) in the evening. You could use a little more phytoestrogen in the evening than first thing in the morning. If you are having hot flashes, I would not worry about taking too much at one time, since hot flashes are telling you that you are severely estrogen or progesterone deficient and you need to address that as quickly as possible.

Hormone Testing

To determine what your hormone levels are, you can do either blood tests or saliva tests. Saliva tests are preferred by Dr. John Lee, who has written several books on menopause and perimenopause.

I strongly recommend you do additional research on hormone issues. I am not a hormone expert and it is important for you to make informed decisions.

Chinese Medicine

Estrogen corresponds to the "yin" in Chinese medicine. It is the cool and moist. As you age, you lose more yin and dozens of symptoms can affect you. The "yang" is the hot and dry, similar to testosterone. You have too little estrogen, relative to your testosterone. You still might need both hormones.

There are several acupuncture points that will balance your hormones. Spleen 6 and Kidney 6 are very commonly used points. Kidney 6 is specific for hot flashes. These points work by making your kidneys stronger so they can keep your hormones in balance. Please see the acupressure chapter for more details.

One herbal formula that is effective for hot flashes is called "Er Zhi Wan." This formula is two herbs, Fructus Ligustri Lucidi and Herba Eclipta. The common names are Ligustrum and Eclipta. The Pin Yin (Chinese) names are Nu Zhen Zi and Han Lian Cao. This formula can be effective on its own to relieve hot flashes.

Chinese herbal formulas such as Er Zhi Wan can be used to treat the underlying imbalance that results in a hormone deficiency. Your acupuncturist can determine which herbal formula is right for you. In some cases, acupuncture and herbs are enough to balance your hormones, without additional supplements.

In Chinese medicine theory, the kidney energy declines as you get older. It is common in China to take Chinese herbal tonics to replenish the kidney energy. This will not only improve your health right now, but it will improve longevity.

Herbal tonics such as He shou wu (fo-ti), Goji berries and American ginseng can be taken to reduce the effects of aging. They are rejuvenating tonics and they can be taken long term. Fo-ti is especially good for longevity enhancement. It replenishes the kidneys, improves hair growth on the head and has been used for fertility for centuries.

Are Phytoestrogens Safe?

These herbs have been used for hundreds of years to treat the symptoms of menopause. All herbs should only be used if you need them. If you take something you do not need, it can cause an imbalance. You can consult with your health care practitioner to discuss what is appropriate for you.

If hormone deficiencies are affecting your sleep, there are many options. Phytoestrogens are one. Acupuncture and herbs are another. Chinese herbs are not known to be estrogenic and are not intended to be used for that. They strengthen the kidneys and help them to produce hormones on their own. These herbs need to be prescribed by a licensed acupuncturist, because each person might need a different formula, depending on her exact diagnosis.

The hormones in phytoestrogen products are not the same as the ones used in pharmaceuticals that are derived from pregnant horse urine.

Hormonal Herbs

There are several herbs to be careful with if you are over 40 or have symptoms of hormone imbalance such as hot flashes:

Rhodiola rosea-This is an energy tonic, but it is too "hot" for women. It can be too strong to use alone if you already have menopause symptoms.

Horny goat weed- men use this for libido. It should only be taken if prescribed by a licensed acupuncturist with a degree in Chinese medicine. The hormonal effects of this herb are very strong. You can quickly have too much testosterone, causing many symptoms such as insomnia, irritability, and facial hair growth.

Panax ginseng- This herb is used in small amounts to boost energy. If you have hot flashes, this can make them worse. Never take this herb as a single herb. An herbalist will be able to give you herbal tonics that do not cause side effects. A thorough diagnosis is needed to determine what is right for you.

Korean ginseng- This herb is too stimulating for most people. It can easily causes excess testosterone in women. I do not recommend this herb for anyone. It should only be used if prescribed.

Eucommia bark-Combined with Cordyceps in Cordyceps Power from Planetary Herbals. This is great for frequent urination and nighttime urination. If you are over 40 and female, be careful how long you take it.

Cordyceps sinensis – If you already have hot flashes, this could make them worse. If you take it a few weeks, it is unlikely to cause a problem. See your acupuncturist for an evaluation if you are female and over 40. In most cases, it should not cause a problem.

Some people take it long term during menopause, with no problems.

None of these supplements should be used by pregnant women unless under the care of a physician.

Hormonal Points:

- See your healthcare practitioner to determine which hormones you need.
- There are many good books that explain hormones in depth. Dr. John Lee has several books, including *What Your Doctor May Not Tell You About Menopause* and *Hormone Balance Made Simple.*
- Each practitioner/author has preferences on testing and dosage. It is always good to go by how you feel also.
- Take only the amount of hormones or phytoestrogen that you need to improve symptoms.
- Progesterone production can decline to near zero at menopause.
- Estrogen levels drop 40 to 60 percent.

There is a lot of disagreement in the medical community about which type of hormone testing is most accurate and which supplements or bio-identical hormones are best. Your health care practitioner can help you make decisions, but it is important to educate yourself.

Chapter 5

Caffeine

It goes without saying that drinking high levels of caffeine before bed can affect your sleep. Some people get by with drinking coffee before bed, but most do not. Over time, you can also become sensitive to things that did not bother you before. In addition to keeping you awake, caffeine alters sleep patterns and can affect how deeply you sleep.

One of the main reasons that caffeine is a problem for some people is that even if you take the caffeine earlier in the day and think it will not affect your sleep, your body might not have been able to excrete the caffeine by the time you want to get to sleep.

Your body needs at least 5 hours to remove half the caffeine you have consumed. Each person has different rates of excretion. Some people take several times as long to remove the caffeine they have consumed. If you drink one cup of coffee that has 200 mg of caffeine, after 5 or more hours, you will still have half that amount or 100 mg in your body. It can take several days to completely excrete all the caffeine you have consumed.

Caffeine Content

Instant Coffee	60-100 mg per cup
Fresh Coffee	80-350 mg per cup
No Doz	100 mg per tablet
5 hour energy	138 mg each
Mountain Dew	54 mg per 12 oz. can
Coca Cola	29 mg per 12 oz. can

If you suddenly reduce your morning caffeine consumption, you can get a headache in the morning. Your body gets used to getting the caffeine at the same time every day and stopping suddenly might be difficult. If you gradually reduce your consumption, the side effects are reduced.

Chapter 6

More Causes of Insomnia

In addition to all the other causes in this book, there are other factors that can affect your sleep.

Multi-vitamin Use Before Bed

Taking multi-vitamins before bed or even in the evening can keep you awake. It is not uncommon for people to take vitamins before bed. Most multi-vitamins have B vitamins in them. These vitamins will boost your energy and keep you awake if taken at night. All vitamins should be taken in the morning or before noon.

Computer and Internet Stimulation

Exposure to electromagnetic radiation and light from monitors affects your brain more than other types of light. Exposure to any type of light in the evening hours can disrupt your sleep, because it is believed to affect your melatonin levels. If you can, turn off your computer monitors in the evening and read a book or magazine to relax. The less artificial light you are exposed to in the evening, the easier it will be to get to sleep.

Food Allergies

Many people have food allergies they are not aware of. Food allergies can cause your adrenal glands to excrete excess adrenaline. Allergic reactions stimulate your body. The most common food allergies are: wheat, oats, corn, all grains, eggs, and gluten. Even gluten free bread can irritate some people. Dairy is also irritating to a lot of people. That includes cheese, milk, sour cream, yogurt.

A good alternative to cow milk is coconut milk. Coconut Dream is a good brand. They also make a dairy free chocolate. Coconut milk is the same consistency as whole cow milk. The chocolate is called Chocolate Dream. Their website is www.tastethedream.com. Coconut oil and milk also boost metabolism and have many other health benefits. A good website for information on dairy free options is www.godairyfree.org.

Coughing or sneezing while eating or after eating are common symptoms of a reaction to what you just ate. Even the urge to clear your throat is a sign your body is making mucus to protect itself from what you ate or drank. Sinus pain is often caused by dairy allergies or sensitivities. Even if you have been allergy tested, that does not completely rule out the possibility of a reaction. No allergy test is definitive. I use the word allergy here, but you can also call it sensitivity.

Bright Lights

If you have an alarm clock that is lit and put it by your head, that light can affect you. It can either keep you up or affect your sleep in other ways. Even if your eyes are closed, your body can sense it. You can also be affected by the sound of some alarm clocks. You can try putting the clock across the room to see if that helps. Pointing the clock away from your head might be necessary. It is a combination of the light and electro-magnetic radiation that can affect you if you are sensitive to it.

Blood Sugar Imbalances

If you have blood sugar balance problems, you can wake in the middle of the night. The Amino acid L-carnitine can be very helpful to balance your blood sugar. Just taking 500 to 1,000 mg in the morning will help balance your blood sugar throughout the day. There are several different types of L-Carnitine. I prefer the Tartrate form for blood sugar issues. I like the Jarrow "Licaps." They are liquid gel carnitine inside of a capsule. If you cannot find that type, any L-carnitine will help balance blood sugar.

Eating Late at Night

If you eat a big meal right before bed, this can affect your sleep. Your stomach wakes up and becomes very active trying to digest your food. Everyone has different tolerance levels to how much they can eat before bed.

Lying on Your Left Side

In Chinese medicine theory, the blood must return to your liver at night. That is why they recommend sleeping on your right side. In modern theory, we know that lying on your left side puts a little more pressure on your heart.

Lying on Your Back

You might find you do not snore if you don't lie on your back. Lying on your back can cause the tongue to obstruct the airway more and lead to snoring. Snoring is often caused by dairy sensitivities. Eating food that you do not tolerate well causes a slight swelling of mucosal tissue in your sinuses and throat. It also causes an increase in mucus production. If you are in doubt, stop all dairy for a few days, even the cream or milk in your coffee, and see if that helps.

Chapter 7

When Pain Keeps You Awake

If you are in pain, you will have a very hard time getting to sleep. There is nothing worse than tossing and turning due to pain.

There are over-the-counter natural remedies that are very effective to treat pain. If given time, these remedies might be enough to completely treat your pain.

Most pain is caused by inflammation. You can have inflamed tendons, nerves, and muscles. If these over-the-counter remedies do not completely fix your pain, please consider acupuncture. There can be many underlying causes for pain that need to be addressed. Acupuncture treats pain by restoring normal circulation. If you have normal circulation, the body can heal itself.

Bromelain

Bromelain is an enzyme that is derived from pineapple. An enzyme is something that dissolves things. If you eat raw pineapple, not canned, you might notice an irritation in your tongue. The irritation is caused by the pineapple dissolving the coating on your tongue. As you chew on it, it eats away the inside of your mouth. Some people are sensitive to this and think they are allergic to it. You might be allergic, or you might just have an irritation. Canned pineapple has been boiled. When the pineapple is boiled, it will not be useful for pain relief. The enzymes are killed when heated.

An alternative to eating raw pineapple is to take Bromelain capsules. When you take this on an empty stomach, the enzymes go into your blood stream and your body uses them to resolve inflammation and break down scar tissue.

When you shop for Bromelain, you want to look at the label and find out how many active units there are. The number of milligrams is irrelevant. Enzymes are measured in *active units*. That will tell you how strong that supplement is. The most common strength is 600 GDU. That is 600 active units. I prefer to take stronger tablets. The one I use is Source Naturals 2,000 GDU per tablet or capsule. This is over 3 times as strong, so you need fewer pills. There are other brands that have 2,000 or 3,000 active units per tablet.

You can take bromelain on an empty stomach when you first get up in the morning, or at any time. Just allow about 30 minutes before you eat or 2 hours after you eat. If you have eaten recently or you eat right after taking Bromelain, it will be used to digest your food. Bromelain is a protease, so it dissolves protein. It is not bad to take it with food, but you will usually need to take more of it to relieve pain.

A lot of people have a hard time remembering the name, bromelain. You can just remember the name "pineapple enzyme," that is often on the label.

The more supplemental enzymes you can take the better. As we age, our body does not make as many digestive enzymes as it does when younger. That is one of the reasons you have more aches and pains as you age. You do not have enough enzymes to digest your food and do cellular repair.

Your body makes enzymes to be used for digestion. Whatever is left over is used to heal damaged tissue. You have cellular damage every day that needs to be repaired. When you eat food that is hard to digest like a lot of animal protein, you might not have enough enzymes to heal yourself.

Ginger Root

Ginger root is a very effective natural pain reliever. It improves digestion, relieves nausea, and stops diarrhea. The secret is to take a high enough dose.

You can buy ginger root in capsules at just about any store. The capsules are raw ginger root that has been chopped up and encapsulated. You will need to take a lot more tablets if you take that type. Don't worry, you will still get the benefit of it, but taking an extract is much stronger.

When you buy herbs, you want to know if you are getting an extract. Herbs are extracted in either water or alcohol. The herb is boiled in water and the liquid from that is dehydrated with the extracted herb put in tablets or capsules. This is about 4 times as strong as the raw herb. When you look at the label, it will tell you how strong it is. 4x for example means that the herb is about 4 times as strong as the raw herb. It is also a lot easier to digest an extract.

You can either just buy ginger root pills and take about 8 of them, or you can buy ginger root extract and take two pills for the same effect. I don't want to make it complicated. You can go down to your local drugstore or any place where supplements are sold and buy some ginger root. If you would like to take fewer pills, my choice is Planetary Herbals Full Spectrum Ginger Extract. Jarrow also makes a good ginger extract. It is four times as strong as taking regular ginger root.

Chapter 8

Andropause/Low Testosterone

Men have a decline in hormone levels as they age, just like women do. They might not have hot flashes as commonly as women do, but their hormones decline, and that can affect their sleep. As you age, your kidney energy declines. This also causes nighttime urination.

A decline in testosterone that affects the libido is a common problem. This is easily solved with herbal remedies. Your body will make more hormones if you strengthen your kidney energy.

Your kidneys get weaker as you age, and that means they make fewer hormones also.

Common symptoms of a kidney deficiency:

- Low back pain
- Waking at night to urinate
- Knee pain
- Frequent urination
- Fatigue
- Insomnia

These symptoms can be treated by acupuncture and Chinese herbs. You can also take over the counter herbs like Cordyceps to strengthen your kidneys.

Horny Goat Weed

The reason I am bringing up safe libido tonics is because so many men these days take herbs to improve their libido and end up causing insomnia by taking herbs that were never intended to be used in that way.

If you have looked for herbal libido tonics, you will have found horny goat weed as a common ingredient. As mentioned in the chapter on menopause, this is not a recommended herb. It is too strong to be taken alone and can quickly cause a hormonal imbalance that causes insomnia. It is not necessary to take herbal tonics that cause a hormonal imbalance to improve libido. The herbs I recommend are cordyceps, goji berries, and American ginseng. Both men and women can take these.

You can quickly cause insomnia by taking herbs like horny goat weed. Other symptoms of excess testosterone are irritability and hot flashes.

The same symptoms caused by excess yang tonics like horny goat weed can be caused by taking too much testosterone prescribed by your medical doctor or bought over the counter. You should be very careful with testosterone. It is easy to develop an imbalance in hormones.

Taking the wrong herbs for your condition can affect your hormones in a week or less in some cases. You will like how you feel when you take these herbs, because they will give you a lot of energy. They are best prescribed by an herbalist.

Libido Tonics

Cordyceps 450 by Planetary Herbals. This is 100% full spectrum Cordyceps extract.

Cordyceps Power, by Planetary Herbals (Cordyceps Mycelia CS-4 Standardized Extract Astragalus Root, Codonopsis Root, Adenophora Root, Eucommia Bark, Eleuthero Root, Bai-Zhu Atractylodes Rhizome and Ginger Root.

Cordyceps Power has cordyceps in and other energy tonics like codonopsis and Siberian ginseng. The herb that affects your kidney and libido the most in this formula is the eucommia bark. Eucommia bark is a yang tonic similar to horny goat weed. Yang is the male and yin is the female, in a loose translation of herbal guidelines. Eucommia is much safer and milder than horny goat weed.

Goji Berries

Goji berries are a liver and kidney tonic. In Chinese herbal lore, men were told to not take a lot of goji berries if they were going on a trip and would be away from their wives a long time.

Goji berries can be taken as a snack. The taste has been described as a cross between a cranberry and a raisin. The best brand in terms of taste is *Dragon Herbs Heaven Mountain*. You can also buy goji berry extract powder and drink it as a tea. Make sure it is the extract, not goji berries ground up into a powder. The traditional Chinese way to make an extract is to boil the herb and make a tea from the liquid. That is much stronger than just using a ground up herb. The best quality is Sun Ten *Gou qi zi*. "Gou qi zi" is the Chinese name for goji berries. Another name for it is Lycium fruit.

If you take goji berries to boost your libido, you will need to take more than the standard dose. To boost energy and improve mood, you can take 2-3 capsules of goji berry extract daily. To boost libido, you might want to double that. A quarter cup of the berries every day as a snack is more than enough to boost libido and energy levels.

Goji berry extract capsules are an easy way to take the berries. The best choices are:

- Planetary Herbals Goji Berry Full Spectrum
- Natural Factors Goji Rich Super Strength Goji Berry
- Nature's Way Standardized Goji Berry

American Ginseng

American ginseng is also a good libido tonic and longevity tonic. The best way to take American ginseng is as an extract. Sun Ten American ginseng extract is very strong. American ginseng is highly prized in China as a tonic for older people. It is more expensive and considered more valuable than Chinese/Panax ginseng.

Hot Flashes in Men

Hot flashes are caused by a deficiency of progesterone and/or estrogen. If you have hot flashes, herbal supplements can treat this.

If you have libido issues, it is very helpful to see an acupuncturist. Several things can cause a low libido. A professional diagnosis is best.

Chapter 9

Are Your Kidneys Waking You Up?

If you can get to sleep, but wake up several times during the night, you might have a syndrome called Kidney Qi or Kidney yang deficiency. This is a diagnosis in Chinese medicine and it has no correlation to a Western medicine diagnosis of kidney problems.

Some common symptoms of a kidney weakness are: Low back pain, weak knees, waking at night to urinate more than once and frequent urination during the day. If you have incontinence when sneezing, you probably have a weakness of your kidney energy.

If your kidneys are weak, you will wake several times to go to the bathroom. Most people think they woke up and since they were already up, they took the opportunity to go to the bathroom. In fact, your weak kidneys woke you up. I've had many discussions with my patients about waking up in the middle of the night. Until their kidneys are stronger, they often do not believe me. It takes about a month to treat this problem. Often, you will start to see an improvement in a week.

It is always good to improve the energy levels of your kidneys. It can also prevent you from being forced to wear a diaper in your old age. Losing control of your bladder is usually caused by weak kidney energy.

Weak kidneys can easily be treated. Chinese herbal remedies such as Cordyceps Sinensis can be used to strengthen your kidneys. Your acupuncturist can prescribe stronger kidney tonics if your kidneys are very weak. Acupuncture is also used to regulate and strengthen your kidney energy.

If you cannot see an acupuncturist, you can try using Cordyceps on your own. It will take longer to recover, but it will work. It normally takes about 30 days to recover from a kidney weakness when you take very strong herbal tonics from an acupuncturist and get acupuncture treatments.

I have used herbs to treat incontinent children and elderly people. I had a patient who was 5 years old and he still wet the bed. His diagnosis was a severe kidney yang deficiency. It took a few months of herbal treatment, but he recovered from this problem. He inherited weak kidney energy from his mother. Do not assume that children are wetting the bed due to emotional issues. Children inherit their kidney strength from their mother. If the mother has weak kidneys, the children can have weak kidneys.

In Chinese medicine theory, the kidneys regulate and hold in the urine. If your kidneys are weak, they cannot perform that function.

The most important acupuncture points for waking at night to urinate and other issues caused by weak kidneys are:

Kidney 3- Treats all aspects of kidney deficiency. Kidney 3 treats fatigue, low back pain, and urinary symptoms. It is effective to treat plantar fasciitis and heel pain. It restores circulation in the foot to relieve pain.

Kidney 6- Treats hot flashes. Excellent for insomnia, it calms you down and nourishes the yin, which is what you lose when you get older. This is one of the most sedative points on the body.

Kidney 7- Strengthens kidneys to resolve low back pain and urinary incontinence. It benefits the "yang." It restores the "fire" of the kidneys. It also restores libido and reduces the retention of excess fluid in the body.

Chinese Medicine Diagnosis

Kidney yang deficiency symptoms include: Aversion to cold, apathy, fatigue, edema in legs (excess fluid), impotence, premature ejaculation, back pain, weak knees.

Kidney yin deficiency symptoms include: Hot flashes, insomnia, hot flashes, night sweats, back pain, dizziness, poor memory, tinnitus, and hair loss.

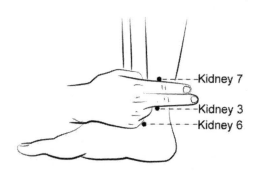

Chapter 10

Valerian Root and Other Sedative Herbs

These herbs should be taken around dinner time or a few hours before bed. It takes time for them to start working. They are mild sedatives. For occasional insomnia, this might be all you need to get to sleep.

Valerian Root- used as a sedative herb for centuries, reduces the time to fall asleep and improves sleep quality. Valerian can stimulate some people, instead of relaxing them. This occurs in about 10% of people. When combined with other sedative herbs, this is less likely to happen.

Hops- calming and sleep inducing, also used for anxiety. Estrogenic and sedative.

Passionflower- mildly sedative. Anti-spasmodic, sedative, anxiety reducing and reduces blood pressure in some. Helps relieve worrying.

Chamomile- Roman or German. Calming, reduces anxiety and tension. Muscle relaxant.

Lemon Balm- relieves tension, anxiety and headaches.

Skullcap- relaxes nerves, sedative.

Sleep Supplements

Chamomile Sleep – Planetary Herbals

This formula combines Western and Chinese herbs to treat the underlying cause of insomnia.

Ingredients: Jujube seed (Zizyphus). Chamomile flower extract. Hops strobiles. Poria sclerotium. American ginseng. Ligusticum, chuan xiong rhizome. Anemarrhena Rhizome. Licorice root

Herbal Notes:

Jujube seed (Zizyphus) is a classic herb used in Chinese medicine to calm the heart energy. It works quickly as a sedative, but it also works on the underlying cause of insomnia.

Poria sclerotium is used in most Chinese herbal tonics. It helps strengthen digestion, improve energy, helps reduce excess fluid in your body, and is also calming.

American ginseng is used as a yin tonic to improve energy but calm you down at the same time. This is especially good for those over 40 or people who are under a lot of stress and feel worn down. This can be taken long term to improve energy levels. It is not as strong as Panax ginseng to improve energy levels, but is often appropriate for those over 50.

Valerian Easy Sleep by Planetary Herbals

Valerian root is a sedative herb that has been used for hundreds of years for anxiety and insomnia. This formula combines valerian root with other herbs for a stronger effect. In most cases, taking herbal combinations is stronger than taking a single herb. You will receive the benefit of all the herbs as well as a synergy of the combination.

Jujube seed, Skullcap, Passionflower leaf and flower, Hops strobili, Wood betony aerial parts, Chamomile flower, Calcium citrate, Magnesium chelate, Dong quai root, Poria sclerotium, Licorice root, Amber resin, American ginseng root, Ginger root, Taurine

If you want to take valerian root as a single herb, the best brands are Nature's way, Solaray and Planetary Herbals Valerian Extract, Full spectrum.

Sound Sleep - Gaia

This is a combination formula in a liquid cap.

Passionflower, Kava kava, American skullcap, Valerian root, California poppy, Blue vervain, Hops strobili, Gotu kola.

Valerian Nighttime- Nature's Way

Valerian root extract 320 mg, Lemon balm extract 160 mg.

Sleep Relax Formula – Natural Factors

Valerian root extract 100 mg, Passion flower extract 50 mg, Hops extract 25 mg, Skullcap 100 mg, Hops, 50 mg.

Revitalizing Sleep Formula – Enzymatic Therapy

Valerian root extract 200 mg, passionflower extract 90mg, L-theanine 50 mg, hops extract 30 mg, wild lettuce extract 18 mg, Jamaica dogwood extract 12 mg, wild lettuce leaf 12 mg.

Remember to take Valerian root and other sedative herbs a few hours before bed. Your body needs time to process the herbs and any supplement taken right before bed can keep you awake.

If you want to take sedative herbs like Valerian root, you will find a lot of formulas have synthetic melatonin included in them. It is very hard to find herbal sleep aids that do not have synthetic melatonin. I even found one sleep formula that had 50 mg of melatonin. That is over 100 times the amount your body makes daily. No one knows the long term effects of taking this.

Another relaxing supplement is chamomile tea. This is not as strong as valerian root and other sedative herbs, but it is a nice tea.

Chamomile is in the ragweed family and might cause sensitivity in allergic people.

Herbal Teas

If you would like to drink herbal teas in the evening, they can be very effective to help you relax. There are dozens of options to choose from. I have excluded some teas that include Rooibos or licorice root, these herbs can be stimulating if taken too late in the evening.

I have chosen several good teas that have a high concentration of the active sleep herbs:

Serene Dream by Octavia Tea

All organic: Valerian, lemon verbena, lemon myrtle, lemon balm, chamomile, lavender, spearmint. All loose teas. I find the loose teas are often stronger than tea in bags.

Organic Lemon Balm Tea by Traditional Medicinals

Organic lemon balm leaf

Organic Chamomile with Lavender by Traditional Medicinals

All organic: Chamomile flower, English lavender, lemon balm leaf

Chapter 11

Melatonin – Is It Safe?

Melatonin is a hormone made in your pineal gland. Your body makes it normally in response to darkness and normal circadian rhythms. Exposure to light reduces melatonin production.

The question is, is it safe to take supplemental synthetic melatonin? In my opinion, it is a bad idea to take melatonin long term to treat insomnia. Insomnia is not caused by a melatonin deficiency. If you treat the underlying cause of your insomnia, you will get to sleep.

Melatonin Facts

About **5-25 mcg** of melatonin are secreted into the blood stream of healthy young and middle-aged men at night time. Notice this is micrograms, not milligrams. The average synthetic melatonin supplement has 5 milligrams.

It is very unlikely you have a melatonin deficiency. I do not know of a test that can be done to determine your levels of melatonin. If you are not deficient in melatonin, should you be taking it in a supplement?

Melatonin is a hormone. It is not a sleep aid. Synthetic melatonin in supplements does not affect your body in the same way as your body's own melatonin.

Synthetic melatonin supplements rapidly increase melatonin levels, while naturally produced melatonin is a gradual build up.

High doses of melatonin have been used as a contraceptive.

Many people who take synthetic melatonin wake up a few hours after going to bed and cannot get back to sleep.

Research on melatonin shows no benefit of taking dosages higher than .25 mg per day. Higher doses are not better, in this case.

Possible side effects of synthetic melatonin

- Headaches
- Nausea
- Drowsiness the next day
- Nightmares
- Abnormal heart rhythms
- High blood pressure
- Confusion
- Difficulty concentrating
- Mood changes
- Fatigue
- Waking at 2 AM, after melatonin levels drop

How Much Melatonin Do You Need?

Your body makes less than one half a milligram at night. Most supplements start at 5 milligrams and go up. If you do not have a melatonin deficiency and you take melatonin as a supplement, what happens? No one knows. That's the problem.

Taking synthetic melatonin to get to sleep is not the same as taking any other sleep supplement. It is a hormone that is used to adjust circadian rhythms. It is not a sleep aid. Taking supplemental hormones might cause health issues that we are not even aware of. If a melatonin deficiency is not the cause of your insomnia, is it a good idea to take it anyway?

You might remember when synthetic estrogen was given automatically to women who had hot flashes or any other menopausal symptoms. After many years of this, it was determined that this can increase the risk of cancer and stroke. Synthetic hormones do not work in your body like natural hormones.

In my opinion, the current usage of synthetic melatonin might end up with a similar ending. We will discover that there are long term effects to taking synthetic melatonin regularly to get to sleep. If you are already on synthetic melatonin, you might have to taper off. Your brain might have stopped making its own supply temporarily.

I am aware that some people will be unhappy with me for saying I do not recommend synthetic melatonin.

As far as I'm concerned, it has a lot of side effects that we know about and some we might not know about for years. Since there are so many other options to treat insomnia naturally, it is not worth the risk to me.

Many medical doctors who at one time recommended synthetic melatonin supplements, have now reversed their position and are warning about high doses and how many times per week you should take it. Most doctors recommend .5 mg per day, only a few times per week, if at all.

Tart Cherries Contain Natural Melatonin

If you are currently taking synthetic melatonin or want to take a healthy alternative, you can try tart cherries.

Montmorency tart cherries contain more melatonin than sweet cherries. Each gram of tart cherries contains up to 13.5 nanograms of natural melatonin.

Tart cherries have the added benefit of treating gout and being a natural pain reliever. You can also try tart cherry juice.

Tart Cherry Supplements

Tart Cherry by Solaray – Fruit *concentrate* with 425 mg per capsule.

Tart Cherry by Solgar – Fruit *extract* with 250 mg of extract per capsule.

Chapter 12

Flower Essences

Flower essences are one of the most effective treatments available for insomnia and other emotional issues. I have a success rate of 90% with Bach Rescue Sleep. Rescue Sleep is a combination of several flower essences that calm you down and stop your mind from racing.

Each flower essence has an energy pattern. It treats certain emotional imbalances. Just like herbs have specific ailments they treat, flowers treat emotional issues. You choose the flower you take based on what emotional issue is affecting you the most at that moment. You can take the flowers either as you need them, or to treat underlying emotional imbalances.

For example, you can use Rescue Sleep for bedtime and Rescue Remedy to deal with stress and anxiety during the day. If you have an underlying depression, you can choose a flower that treats the kind of depression you have. You will benefit from the flower, regardless if you choose the correct one. Everyone could benefit from the flowers, so there is no loss in taking a variety.

I have to admit that I did not believe flower essences worked before I tried them, so I can understand the skepticism of some people. Once you try them, you will be a believer. These remedies are extracted with water, but preserved with alcohol. So, if you are alcohol sensitive, please be aware of this. There are some flower essences that are preserved with glycerin. They are alcohol free. There are also Rescue Remedy Sleep Liquid melts that are in tablet form.

Dr. Edward Bach

Dr. Edward Bach was a homeopathic doctor in London in the early 1900s. He believed that the majority of his patients were affected by emotional issues. In fact, he felt most diseases were emotionally caused. He did research and developed his own remedies for emotional imbalances.

He left his busy London practice and went to the English countryside and tried different flowers on himself. Each flower has an emotion associated with it. Just as each herb has diseases it treats, so does each flower.

How to take Bach flower remedies

You can spray the flowers directly into your mouth several times or use a dropper. This provides an immediate effect. You can also put the flowers in your drinking water. This is how you use the flowers for a longer lasting and deeper treatment. Each flower can be taken as long as needed. There are no negative side effects. In fact, it is best to focus on the positive benefits of the flowers, rather than the negative ones. For example, taking the Impatiens essence will give you more patience. Rather than saying you are taking it because you are impatient, you take it to become more patient.

Bach Rescue Sleep can be kept by your bed. You can take it before you go to bed and if you wake up in the middle of the night. It is not physically sedating, it just relaxes your mind so much that you might feel like it is. Especially in the beginning, I would take the Rescue Sleep right before bed. The first few times you take it, you will feel a big difference.

When you take the flowers, you are working for an immediate effect, but you also receive a long term effect. Taking Bach Rescue Sleep at night will make you calmer the next day. It helps to calm your mind down. You can take Bach Rescue Remedy during the day to deal with anxiety and stress.

Bach Rescue Sleep Remedy

Bach Rescue Sleep is a combination of flower essences that is used to relieve stress and anxiety. It calms your mind down and stops repetitive thoughts. You can spray two to three times in your mouth about 30 minutes before you want to go to sleep. You can repeat as often as necessary. You might feel like you have taken a sedative, since the relaxation effect is so strong. There is no sedative. You are only feeling relaxed and calm.

The **Bach Rescue Sleep** remedy is made of the following flower essences:

White Chestnut: To help ease restless mind.
Star of Bethlehem: For trauma and shock.
Clematis: For the tendency to "pass out," and unconsciousness, being 'far away' and not present mentally.
Cherry Plum: Fear of mind giving way, verge of breakdown, anger.
Impatiens: For irritability, tension, and fidgety.
Rock Rose: For frozen terror and panic.

I have tried Bach Rescue Sleep on many patients. It is not a sedative, but it feels like one to most people. It calms your mind and helps you stop repetitive thoughts. It helps you relax and get your mind off things. You will not be drowsy in the morning from this. Also, the emotional relaxation will not only help you sleep, but it will help you to be calmer throughout the day. It has a cumulative effect.

For sleep, you can spray the Rescue Sleep in your mouth right before bed. If you keep it on the nightstand, you can use it as needed. Try three sprays before bed. In most cases, one dose is enough. Taking Rescue Sleep remedy before bed will also improve your stress level during the day.

Bach Rescue Remedy

Bach Rescue Remedy is for daytime use, for stress, and anxiety.

You can spray some in your mouth and also put some in your drinking water. When you put it directly in your mouth, it works faster. When you put some in a glass of water and drink it, the effect is deeper. That is why it is good to do both. I recommend this to my patients for anxiety and panic attacks as well as stress.

The official Bach flower site has a lot of free information and includes case study information: www.bachcentre.com.

From studying flower essences, you can understand emotional issues better. Sometimes you do not recognize which emotional issue you have until you analyze the flower essences to determine which one is right for you. The flower essence books will explain the flowers in more detail. The best book for this is *Bach Flower Therapy, Theory and Practice* by Mechthild Scheffer.

Bach Flower Essences

Agrimony - mental torture behind a cheerful face. Denial of emotional pain, addiction behaviors.

Aspen - fear of unknown things. Anxiety, fear, and foreboding.

Beech – intolerance. Critical attitude, perfectionist, and hypersensitive.

Centaury - the inability to say 'no'. Weak willed. Co-dependency issues.

Cerato - lack of trust in one's own decisions. Depend too much on advice from other people.

Cherry Plum - fear of the mind giving way. Emotional breakdown. Eating disorders due to losing control.

Chestnut Bud - failure to learn from mistakes. Addiction, breaking bad habits.

Chicory - selfish, possessive love. Demanding and needy behavior. Self-centered.

Clematis - dreaming of the future without working in the present. Having frequent daydreams to avoid current problems. Escapism.

Crab Apple--the cleansing remedy, also for self-hatred. Feeling imperfect. Feeling ashamed of yourself.

Elm--overwhelmed by responsibility. Feeling exhausted.

Gentian--discouragement after a setback. Doubt.

Gorse--hopelessness and despair. Discouragement, pessimism.

Heather--self-centeredness and self-concern. Seeking attention and sympathy.

Holly--hatred, envy, and jealousy. Positive aspect: opens the heart to love.

Honeysuckle--living in the past. Unwilling to face the future.

Hornbeam--procrastination, tiredness at the thought of doing something. Feeling overwhelmed.

Impatiens--impatience. Irritable, tense, intolerant, stressed.

Larch--lack of confidence. Expect to fail.

Mimulus--fear of known things. Anxiety and escapism.

Mustard--deep gloom for no reason. Despair and depression.

Oak--the plodder who keeps going past the point of exhaustion. Overwhelm.

Olive--exhaustion following mental or physical effort. Complete exhaustion.

Pine--guilt. Self-criticism. Co-dependence.

Red Chestnut--over-concern for the welfare of loved ones. Negative worry for others.

Rock Rose--terror and fright. Fear of death.

Rock Water--self-denial, rigidity and self-repression. Inability to enjoy life, dogmatic.

Scleranthus--inability to choose between alternatives. Indecision between two options.

Star of Bethlehem--shock. Trauma. Deeply restorative and soothing remedy.

Sweet Chestnut--Extreme mental anguish, when everything has been tried and there is no light left. Deep depression and despondency. "Dark night of the soul."

Vervain--over-enthusiasm. Overbearing. Nervous exhaustion.

Vine--dominance and inflexibility. Strong willed. Aggressive.

Walnut--protection from change and unwanted influences. Affected by beliefs that hold you back.

Water Violet--pride and aloofness. Appearing distant.

White Chestnut--unwanted thoughts and mental arguments. Repetitive thoughts. Mind racing.

Wild Oat--uncertainty over one's direction in life. Lack of focus. Helps you find your life's mission.

Wild Rose--drifting, resignation, apathy. Giving up on life.

Willow--self-pity and resentment. Bitterness. Feeling like a victim.

There are hundreds of flower essences available. Most people feel they could take all of them at one time or another. The top selling flower essences in my office are Bach Rescue Sleep, Rescue Remedy, Sweet Chestnut for depression, Impatiens for stress, Cherry plum for feeling like you are going to lose your mind and an aide for binge eating.

FES - Flower Essence Services

FES stands for Flower Essences Services. This company is based in California and makes flower essences from American flowers. They also do research on flower essences. They can be found at www.fesflowers.com.

A few FES flower essences that you might find helpful:

Madia – Easily distracted, inability to concentrate.

Nicotiana – Numbing of emotions with substances. For tobacco or nicotine addiction. My patients find this very helpful to help them stop smoking. I combine it with Chinese herbs like Bupleurum D and acupuncture to relieve stress. I start herbs and acupuncture for stress a few weeks before the patient tries to quit. This eases the transition with less anxiety.

Peppermint – Mental lethargy, feeling sluggish. Makes you more alert and focused. Peppermint essential oil is also good for this.

Chamomile- Easily upset, moody, irritable. Good for Insomnia.

Lavender – Nervous, over-stimulated, stressed, and irritable.

Cayenne- Stagnation, inability to move forward to change.

Evening primrose – Feeling rejected, unwanted. Repressed, painful childhood.

Flourish Formulas from FES

Flourish flower essences are a line of combination flower essences from the FES company. These products are combinations of different flowers. Each remedy has several flowers that treat the same emotional imbalance. For example, the Fear-Less formula has several flowers that treat fear. Using a variety of flowers can be more effective than just using one flower. The Bach Rescue Remedy is an example of this. The flowers are combined to enhance the effect of the others. The Flourish formulas come in a spray bottle. These formulas are very effective.

Detailed information on each flower in this line is available at www.fesflowers.com/flourish.htm.

These flower remedies are not for sleep, but they are very popular, so I'm including them.

Activ 8 – Eight flowers to inspire you to action. Overcome procrastination. Flower essences: Blackberry, cayenne, red penstemon, red larkspur, sunflower, madia, dandelion, blazing star.

Fear-Less – Fear, anxiety and panic. Flower essences: Red clover, mountain pride, California Valerian, Oregon grape, mimulus, rock rose, green rose.

Illumine – Depression and discouragement. Flower essences: Mustard, St. John's wort, borage, explorers gentian, pine.

Mind-full – Mental clarity, focus and concentration. Flower essences: Peppermint, lemon, morning glory, nasturtium, cosmos, Shasta daisy, Rabbitbrush, and madia.

The website for FES is www.fesflowers.com. You can buy your essences from their site and many other supplement sites. Bach flower essences are available at most health food stores. Brands other than Bach are not as easy to find at stores, but Amazon carries a big selection.

Flower Essences for Children

Bach flower essences also have formulas for children. The flowers are not preserved in alcohol and include **Rescue Remedy**, **Daydream**, and **Confidence**. These formulas are preserved with glycerin instead of alcohol. Although there is not enough alcohol to be contraindicated for children, the formulas preserved in glycerin are a good option. These can also be used by alcohol sensitive people.

For more information on flower essences, check out www.Nelsonsnaturalworld.com, www.BachCentre.com, www.fesflowers.com.

These remedies can also be used on pets and children. Children are especially responsive. You can either put a drop in their water bottle or spray some on their hands or wrist. I've wanted many times to be able to spritz some Rescue Remedy on babies on airplane trips. Unfortunately, most people do not know about the flowers and would probably not react well to my suggestion.

Flower Essence Products

Bach Rescue Sleep- use before bed for sleep

Bach Rescue Remedy- for stress and anxiety

Bach Rescue Energy – for fatigue

Bach Rescue Pastille- Black Currant – non-alcoholic

Rescue Remedy Cream- non-alcoholic

Rescue Sleep liquid melts – non-alcoholic

Pet Rescue Remedy

Kids Rescue Remedy – non-alcoholic

Creature Comforters Six Pet Blends – a line made for pets. This line is carried by Amazon. They have a lot of information on how to use flower essences for your pets. www.CreatureComforters.co.uk.

Chapter 13

Amino Acids

Amino acids are components of protein. You can buy amino acids in pill form. Your body uses amino acids to make brain neurotransmitters.

Amino Acid Notes:

- Do not take long term.
- Take a small dose in the beginning, a higher dosage is not more effective.
- If dosage is too high, this is just as bad as not having enough.
- Do not take amino acids if you are taking medications such as SSRIs. These drugs make your brain recycle serotonin. If you take a supplement that increases serotonin, you can have too much serotonin.
- If you take amino acids, do not combine them with other sleep products.
- If you take amino acids and feel no effect, it simply means you did not need them.

Eighty percent of your body's serotonin is made in your intestines. There is evidence that a lack of the good probiotics in your intestines reduces the amount of the feel good brain neurotransmitters.

Probiotics

Our good bacteria are constantly assaulted by the food and water we eat and drink.

My personal choice for probiotics is Garden of Life *Primal Defense* and Dr. Ohhira's brand called *Essential Formulas*. Other good brands are Jarrow *EPS* and Renew Life *Ultimate Care*, which has 50 billion live cultures per capsule.

Each person will respond differently to probiotics. You could take one product and not notice a difference and take another and start feeling better. We all need to take probiotics on a regular basis for digestive health. Many things in our diets destroy the good bacteria in our intestines. This sets us up for health problems later on.

If you are taking medication that affects your serotonin levels as SSRI, selective serotonin reuptake inhibitors, you should not take amino acids. The medication prevents your body from excreting the serotonin once it has been used. Your brain continues to recycle it. If you take amino acids in this situation, you can have an excess of serotonin, which is just as bad as too little. Since amino acids are just one of many natural sleep aids, it is not worth taking a chance.

If you are on any type of medication, I would skip the amino acids. Amino acids can strongly affect brain chemistry. The other supplements in this book are gentler in action.

The most commonly used amino acids used to relax or sleep are: Theanine, tryptophan, GABA and 5-htp.

5-HTP

5-htp is used to improve serotonin levels. Too much 5htp can make you nauseous. Taking more is not better with amino acids. It is better to start with 50 mg capsules. It can be taken in the morning. 5-htp is also used for food cravings and depression.

L-Tryptophan

L-Tryptophan is a precursor to serotonin. Your body can use it to make both serotonin and melatonin.

GABA

Gamma-aminobutyric acid (GABA), a neurotransmitter involved in inhibition and stress relief. This amino acid is used for stress and anxiety.

Theanine

Theanine is derived from green tea. It is relaxing and relieves anxiety. It increases serotonin and dopamine production.

Amino Acid Recommendations

I do not recommend amino acids as a first line treatment for insomnia. They affect brain chemistry more than the other products recommended and it is possible to take too much, causing side effects.

If you decide to try them, take the smallest dose possible and do not take every day or long term.

Chapter 14

Essential Oils

Essential oils such as lavender and ylang ylang can be used to improve relaxation and sleep. They work by acting directly on the brain to induce relaxation.

The best essential oils for sleep are: Lavender, valerian, neroli, clary sage, vetiver, Roman chamomile, patchouli, ylang ylang and Jasmine. Each aromatherapist will have favorites. The easiest way to use essential oils for sleep is to buy a blend. This will give you the benefits of several oils.

When shopping for essential oil, be sure the label says "pure essential oil," otherwise you can get oil that has been diluted with another type of oil such as almond oil.

For sleep and relaxation, lavender oil is the most effective essential oil. The easiest way to use it is to put a few drops on your wrists or to put a few drops in a small plate next to your bed.

Bath products that are lavender scented rarely have the lavender essential oil in them. They often use lavender fragrance, which will not have the same effect.

Essential Oil Products

Pillow Potion Mist- Aura Cacia

Lavender, sweet orange, hops, patchouli, yarrow, German chamomile

Lavender Mist by Aura Cacia

Lavender essential oil

Elixir of Dreams Pillow Mist by Earth Therapeutics – Lavender and valerian essential oil blend to spray on your pillow.

Calming Lavender Mineral Bath – Aura Cacia

Aura Cacia makes a big variety of essential oil products, including blends. www.auracacia.com.

California Baby Aromatherapy Spritzer, Overtired and Cranky formula.

Roman chamomile, tangerine, orange.

I like this line by California Baby, they have a lot of organic aromatherapy products for babies. They are at www.californiababy.com.

Epsom Salts Bath with Essential Oil

A bath of Epsom salts, which is magnesium sulfate, can be combined with a drop of essential oils. The Epsom salts relax the muscles. If you don't want to take a full bath, soaking your feet in warm water with Epsom salts and essential oils is a good way to get the benefit. Soaking your feet in warm water is relaxing because it pulls energy to your feet and away from your head.

Chapter 15

White Noise

If you have too much noise around you at night, or are just a light sleeper, you might try white noise. There are machines that make white noise, which cancels out the other sounds that might keep you awake. You can also try a CD with rainfall on it. Rain sounds can be very relaxing.

The trick is to find a CD that does not have thunder on it. **Rain for sleeping and relaxation** by Joe Baker is a good one. You can play this CD on a continual loop on your CD player. If you live on a busy street or have noisy neighbors, this is a good option. www.sleepylittlebaby.com.

Hearos Ear Plugs Xtreme Protection- Some people have success with ear plugs. You can buy disposable ear plugs to block out noise. www.hearos.com.

Sleep phones are an option. They are in a headband that covers your ears. This will help to block out noise, as well as play music to relax you. www.sleepphones.com.

Delta Sleep System from Dr. Jeffrey Thompson is a very relaxing CD. I have used several of his CDs in my office and my patients find them relaxing. www.neuroacoustic.com.

Ecotones Sound + Sleep Machine by Adaptive Sound Technologies -This product has 10 natural sound recordings to choose from. www.soundofsleep.com

HoMedics Sound Spa Relaxation Machine with 6 Nature Sounds by Homedics. www.homedics.com.

Marpac Dohm-DS Dual Speed Sound Conditioner by Marpac. www.marpac.com.

Chapter 16

Treating the Cause of Insomnia

How Energy Tonic Herbs Can Help

If you have occasional insomnia, it is often enough to take Valerian root, flower essences, and the other things listed in this book. However, if you have chronic insomnia, you will need to treat the underlying cause.

As an acupuncturist, I have never failed to successfully treat insomnia if the patient persevered and did what was needed, i.e., Chinese herbs and acupuncture. All acupuncturists are pain relief and insomnia experts, because we treat them all day, every day.

The number of treatments you need is determined by how many things you have wrong with you. Insomnia can be the result of many different diagnoses. You might have several things causing your insomnia. In many cases, a 4 to 6 week commitment is all that is needed. Most patients start sleeping better the first week of treatment.

If you are not able to get acupuncture, there are herbs you can take over the counter that will treat fatigue. In order to be healthy, you have to have good digestion, good sleep, and good energy levels. This is where sleep sedatives fail, whether they are herbal or pharmaceutical. The underlying cause has to be treated, if you want to have complete relief from insomnia.

Astragalus and Codonopsis

Astragalus and Codonopsis are Chinese herbs that improve energy levels and digestion. These herbs are gentle enough to be used for children. In China, raw Astragalus is boiled in soups to improve the immune systems and digestion of children. You can buy astragalus extract powder and make it into a tea and/or put it in food like mashed potatoes.

Extracted herbs are 3-4 times as strong as raw herbs. They are made by boiling the raw herbs in water and dehydrating the liquid from that to make the tablets. The herbs are much easier to absorb and you can take fewer pills.

When looking for herbal extracts, it is often necessary to use the Chinese name. The herbs made by companies that make herbs for acupuncturists, like Sun Ten, make the best herbal extracts you can buy. Astragalus is called "Huang Qi", which means yellow energy. This refers to the energy you get from taking it. Codonopsis is called "Dang Shen". www.acuatlanta.net carries the Sun Ten brand.

Panax Ginseng

Panax ginseng is used in Chinese herbal medicine to make the heart energy stronger. The heart has more energy, so it pumps harder. If you have high blood pressure, you should seek the care of a licensed herbalist. It can also affect you hormonally. The most common dosage of ginseng in formulas is only 10%, and a larger dose is not necessary. There are many tonic herbs that can improve your energy levels. Ginseng is just the most famous tonic herb.

Planetary Herbals has a line of over-the-counter Chinese herbal tonics that include Codonopsis and Astragalus extract. I mention this company a lot because they have high quality products that are formulated by Michael Tierra, a famous herbalist. He has several books about herbs, including *"The Way of Chinese Herbs."* If you would like to know more about Chinese herbs and how they can improve your health, this book is a good resource.

In addition to taking Astragalus or Codonopsis, there are a few over the counter herbal formulas that will improve energy and digestion.

Ginseng Elixir- Astragalus Root, licorice root, bupleurum root, Chinese cimicifuga rhizome, molasses, atractylodes, jujube, dong quai root extract, dong quai root and ginger root.

Ginseng Revitalizer – Dong Quai root, atractylodes, Codonopsis, Asian Ginseng (Panax or Chinese ginseng), Fo-ti root, licorice root, astragalus root, eleuthero root, Tienchi Ginseng root, American ginseng root, ginger root, Eleuthero root extract, poria and Asian Ginseng root extract.

Cordyceps sinensis is a kidney, lung and heart tonic. It can be used long term by most people to improve energy levels.

Cordyceps 450, Full Spectrum- 100% Cordyceps sinensis

Cordyceps Power – Cordyceps sinensis, astragalus, Codonopsis root, adenophora root, eucommia bark, eleuthero root, atractylodes, and ginger root.

Taking even a low dose of Chinese herbal tonics is an effective way to improve your energy levels and sleep. These formulas are based on classic herbal remedies that have been used for years to build energy.

If you can get acupuncture, you will recover much more quickly, because your herbal formula will be prescribed for you based on your diagnosis. If you cannot, then taking herbal energy tonics will improve your overall health. They should be taken before 6pm. They can be taken with food.

Chapter 17

Sleep Aids for Kids

For occasional sleep problems, kids can take things like chamomile tea, flower essences, and have gentle acupressure on their Heart 7 and Pericardium 6 points.

When doing acupressure on children, remember that their acupuncture points are located using their measurements, not yours. Use their fingers to measure up from the wrist for Pericardium 6.

There are several good herbal formulas designed for kids.

Calm Child Herbal Syrup by Planetary Herbals

Ingredients: Chamomile Flower, Jujube Seed, Hawthorn Berry, Catnip Aerial Parts, Lemon Balm Aerial Parts, Long Pepper Fruit, Licorice Root, Amla Fruit, Magnesium Taurinate, Calcium Carbonate, Gotu Kola Aerial Parts, and essential oils

Lemon balm and chamomile are gentle relaxation aids

Chinese Zizyphus, gotu kola, amla and hawthorn berry are tonics. Zizyphus is used to calm the heart, gotu kola is effective for anxiety and stress.

Quiet Kids Liquid by Erba Vita

Ingredients: Linden (*Tilia platyphyllus*) (inflorescence), Lemon Balm (*Melissa officinalis*) (leaves), Chamomile (*Matricaria chamomile*) (flowers), Passionflower extract (*Passiflora incarnata*), (aerial part) [standardized to 2% (1 mg), total flavonoids expressed as vitexin], Sweet Orange extract (*Citrus sinensis*) (flowers), English Lavender (*Lavandula officinalis*) (flowers)

Chamomile Calm by Herbs for Kids

Proprietary Blend: An extract of Wood Betony, Chamomile flowers, Fennel seed, Hops strobiles, and Catnip herb.

Hylands Calms Forte for Kids

Homeopathic remedy

Just for Kids, Organic Nighty Night Tea by Traditional Medicinals

Ingredients: Organic linden flower, organic chamomile flower, organic hibiscus flower.

This product is cute, with an owl on the box. It should appeal to kids to have their own tea to drink in the evening.

White Noise for Baby:

mybaby HoMedics SoundSpa On-The-Go

There are other products marketed for use on kids. Some of them contained Theanine. Theanine is an amino acid that helps to calm your brain. I don't have a problem with adults using this, but I do not recommend amino acids for kids. Amino acids should not be taken long term. It is unlikely to be a problem, but children are very sensitive and herbal tonics such as chamomile should be enough.

These children's sleep aids could also be used by adults. Liquid herbs are absorbed faster than tablets or capsules.

Chapter 18

Acupressure

How to Treat Yourself

Acupressure techniques:

- Use a mini or micro massager
- Press or rub firmly with your fingers

Acupressure is the activation of the acupuncture points by either pressing on them or otherwise stimulating them. You can press firmly for about 5 minutes. Sometimes you feel the effect quickly, other times you feel something in an hour. It depends on the point and what you are trying to achieve.

Some acupuncture points are appropriate and effective as acupressure points. Even if you do not feel an effect, that does not mean it is not working. The points perform specific functions when stimulated. It is your response that varies. Each person has a different level of sensitivity.

Getting the Qi

"Getting the Qi" is an expression used by acupuncturists to describe when the point has been activated. The sensations include numbness, tingling, itching, and swelling. An itchy or tingling sensation is the most common and easy to feel.

A feeling of numbness or achiness is more often felt in stronger acupuncture points such as Stomach 36, by the knee. If you are very tired, you might not feel anything at all for a while. In order to feel something, you must have energy. Most people feel something the first or second time, but if you are exhausted, your energy will need to be built up.

Pericardium 6 is used for nausea, heart palpitations, and insomnia. It works by regulating and calming your heart and stomach. It opens up circulation in the chest.

Acupressure wrist bands are popular with pregnant women to treat morning sickness. These bands apply gentle pressure. Sea Band is one brand. You can also try these bands for insomnia. The point Pericardium 6 is used for insomnia.

If these wrist bands are not strong enough to stop morning sickness, you can try acupuncture. The cause of morning sickness is not always the same thing in everyone. Your acupuncturist can determine the cause of your morning sickness.

When you get acupuncture for insomnia, a variety of points will be done that improve sleep. Acupuncture works on the underlying issues to resolve insomnia completely.

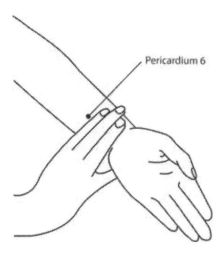

Pericardium 6

Pericardium 6 is found by placing three fingers together and measuring from the wrist crease. The point is between the tendons, but with magnets, it is not so important to be exactly on the point. Each acupuncture point has a range in which it is effective. In other words, *a diameter of about a dime or nickel around where the point is will be effective.* Do not be concerned about being precise in your point location. Just get as close as you can. There are many

YouTube videos showing how to locate acupuncture points.

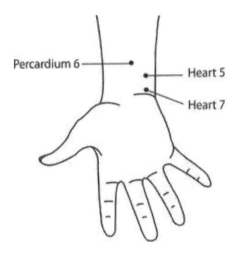

Shown in this image are also Heart 5 and 7. Heart 5 is used to regulate the heart rhythm and Heart 7 is used to calm the heart, which treats anxiety and insomnia. You can press on these points also.

There are many points that are very effective for insomnia. Your diagnosis will determine which points are used. Pericardium 6 is useful for insomnia, nausea, stomach problems, acid reflux, and morning sickness. It regulates digestion and opens up the chest area. It regulates the heart energy and can relieve some types of chest pain, by improving circulation in the chest.

By pressing these points for about 5 minutes, you will help your body to calm down. These points are used by acupuncturists on the majority of patients. The reason they are used so often is that they treat many things. You could just do those acupuncture points and get good results on a variety of health concerns.

A very effective way to do acupressure is with a mini massager. You can buy them for about $10. The best type to use has 3-4 different removable heads. They are marketed to treat diabetic neuropathy and scars. The attachment that has 20 or so prongs on it is the strongest for acupressure. Use the massager for about 5 minutes on each point, on both sides of the body. Treat Pericardium 6 on the left and right wrist. Treat Heart 7 on the left and right wrist. You can spend a few minutes on each, alternating between them.

When you get acupuncture, the needles are usually left in for 20-30 minutes. If 5 minutes of acupressure does not get results, you can do it longer.

Sammons Preston Rolyan makes a mini massager that has the appropriate attachments. I provide a list of other brands and links to buy them on my main site, www.AcupunctureExplained.com. Since this product is used for things other than acupressure, I do not want to recommend more brands in this book. I will keep the page for acupressure updated with new products as

I find them. I will also keep book updates available in
the section for this book.

Chapter 19

Acupuncture

– Is It a Cure for Insomnia?

The most common question acupuncturists get is, "Can acupuncture help...?" The answer is almost always "Yes." Acupuncture has been used as the primary form of medicine in China for over 2,000 years. It is used to treat just about any ailment you might have. It treats you on a holistic level. That means it treats the whole person, not the symptom.

In order to understand how acupuncture can help you, you have to understand how we diagnose disease. We do not use the Western medicine method of diagnosis. For example, if you have fatigue, we do not diagnose you with fatigue. We would get to the root of your fatigue and find out which organ system is out of balance. There are many syndromes that can cause fatigue. Once we have a diagnosis, we can treat the underlying cause.

When you get acupuncture, you can have many ailments treated at the same time. It would be impossible for you to get an acupuncture treatment for back pain that would not also treat your other ailments, because we treat the whole person. Your body heals itself when you give it what it needs. Your body knows what healthy is. It is programmed into your DNA.

When you get acupuncture, you will notice how relaxed you feel. Many people fall asleep when they get acupuncture. It helps to calm your body down and it treats the underlying causes of insomnia. Most people feel better after their first acupuncture session. They feel relaxed. There is always an initial fear or tension about getting acupuncture. After the first needle, you will see how harmless it is and you will be able to relax.

If you decide acupuncture is not for you, acupressure is a good option. Your acupuncturist will be glad to help you find the points and you can also get a prescription for Chinese herbs. Do not let a fear of needles stop you from getting help.

Some common questions people have about acupuncture are:

1. Does it hurt?
2. Will I have to go forever?
3. How many treatments will I need?
4. Do you re-use needles?
5. How big are the needles?
6. How does it feel?
7. Is it safe?
8. How long does it take to see results?
9. How long is each visit?
10. Do I do anything special before my visit?
11. Do you have a degree in this?
12. How often do I get acupuncture?
13. Should I stop my medications when I start acupuncture?
14. How much does acupuncture cost?
15. Does insurance pay for acupuncture?
16. Do I have to believe in it for it to work?
17. When will I start to feel better?
18. What about the placebo effect?
19. What should I expect on my first visit?
20. What about all those images of people with needles in their faces?
21. Do you bleed?
22. How do you find the acupuncture points?

Does it hurt?

Acupuncture needles are hair-fine. They are not like sewing needles or hypodermic needles that are used to give injections. Most people barely feel them. After inserting the first needle, often patients will ask me when I am going to insert it. They did not feel anything.

Each acupuncture point has a different probability of sensitivity. For example, points on the hands or feet are more likely to be sensitive than the arms or legs. That said, we are careful when we treat you to minimize your discomfort.

Will I have to go forever? How many treatments will I need?

You will need to get a series of treatments to completely recover. Your overall health will usually determine how long you get care. If you are fairly healthy, eat well and exercise, you could get well very fast, within a few weeks.

Unfortunately, most people only consider acupuncture after they have been sick a long time and have exhausted every other option. This often means that there are many ailments to address and the level of fatigue must be addressed. If you are exhausted, we will address your energy levels. There is no way to be completely healthy if you have no energy. Your body needs a good level of energy to function properly. We also always address sleep issues. You will not heal if you cannot sleep at night.

You should plan on getting care at least for a month. Although you will start to feel better soon, you will not be completely well. Most patients feel so well after a month, that they say they have not felt so good in years. They had literally forgotten what healthy feels like.

I have had a few people say that they felt tired after acupuncture. They feel tired because they have not felt so relaxed in a long time. They don't even know what it feels like to be relaxed. It is one of the most profound feelings of relaxation you can experience.

Your acupuncturist will work with you. If it is not in your budget to get acupuncture every week, you can work out an arrangement to come in as often as you can. It will take a little longer if you don't come in weekly, but you will still get better.

Do you re-use needles?

Acupuncturists do not re-use needles. Disposable needles cost between five to ten cents each, depending on the brand. Needles would have to be sterilized in an auto-clave and it would not be worth the trouble. After each use, the needles are disposed of in a sharps container, just like in other medical offices.

How big are the needles?

The needles are the size of your hair. The most common gauges are 34, 36, and 38. The most common length used is one inch. Needles range in size from press tacks up to 3 inches. The half inch size is also popular for points on the face and ears.

How does it feel?

You often will not feel the needle go in. If you feel it, it is a slight "ping" feeling. After the needle is inserted, you should not feel discomfort. "Getting the Qi" is when you start to feel the stimulation in the acupuncture point. A few minutes after the needle is inserted you might feel different sensations.

Numbness, tingling, itching, swelling, and aching can occur. The most common is tingling. These sensations tell you the acupuncture point has been activated. After the needles are in for 20 to 30 minutes, you might feel a slight numbness. This is a very good sign. It shows you have a good energy level and the acupuncture treatment has been strong for you.

You have to have very good energy levels to feel numbness. Most people just feel a slight tingling in the beginning. After you have had acupuncture for about a month, your energy levels are improved and you will feel stronger sensations during your session.

Is it safe?

It is important to see a licensed acupuncturist. To get an acupuncture license, you need three to four years of acupuncture school and a Master's degree in Oriental medicine.

Acupuncturists learn over 400 acupuncture point locations, how deep to needle each point, the angle of needle insertion and many other things. For example, when treating the back, we do not insert the needle straight in, it is inserted at an angle.

In order to earn a Master of Science degree in Oriental Medicine, you need to learn about 400 acupuncture points, their indications, contraindications, needle depth, needle angle, and how to combine different points for best effect. Other types of practitioners are allowed to insert acupuncture needles, but if they do not have an advanced degree in Chinese medicine, you are not getting the same benefit.

How long does it take to see results?

The second visit is when you normally start feeling the strongest effect. You will feel something the first visit, but your body will respond faster after the meridians have been activated. Your acupuncturist will be able to give you an educated guess on how long it will take you to get better. We treat the whole body, so many ailments can be treated at the same time.

How long is each visit?

Your first visit will take a little longer than follow-up visits. We ask questions, look at your tongue, and take a thorough medical history. After the needles are inserted, you will relax on the table for 20 to 30 minutes.

Do I do anything special before my visit?

It is best to have a light snack before you get acupuncture. If you are starving and get acupuncture, it will not be as strong. Your body needs food to make energy. Just a bite of something will help you relax better also.

Do acupuncturists get a degree?

A Master's degree in Oriental medicine is the standard in America. N.C.C.A.O.M (National Certification Commission for Acupuncture and Oriental Medicine) accredits and tests acupuncturists. You must pass a standardized test for acupuncture point location, Chinese medicine diagnosis and Chinese herbal medicine to be certified.

Once you are certified and graduate from school, you apply for a state license. Each state has different names for licensed acupuncturists, the most common is L.Ac., for Licensed Acupuncturist. In New Mexico, the title D.O.M. is used. This is Doctor of Oriental

Medicine. In Rhode Island, it is Doctor of Acupuncture, D.A. If your acupuncturist has practiced prior to the time that acupuncture schools were open in America, they might not have a Master's degree. M.S.O.M., is Master of Science, Oriental Medicine.

Different schools offer different degrees. M.S.T.O.M is Master of Science in Traditional Oriental Medicine. M.S.A.O.M is Master of Science in Acupuncture and Oriental Medicine. M.Ac.O.M is Master of Acupuncture and Oriental Medicine.

The curriculum for Acupuncture school includes classes in Western medicine. We learn basic symptoms and treatments. We do not prescribe pharmaceutical drugs. Most acupuncturists will prescribe Chinese herbs and other supplements to speed healing.

If you would like to check out the curriculum, the school I attended is at www.aoma.edu. You might find it interesting to see the depth of education you receive in acupuncture school.

How often do I get acupuncture?

Once or twice a week is the most common frequency. The more often you get care, the faster you get better. In China, a series of daily treatments is given. Each series is usually ten treatments, after that a re-evaluation is given. In the West, it is common to go weekly. If you cannot go every week, you can go every other week and take herbs. Your acupuncturist will work with you on your budget and help you recover as quickly as possible.

Even if you can only get acupuncture once a month, you will still get a benefit and you can take Chinese herbs in between sessions to treat your ailments.

Should I stop my medications when I start acupuncture?

Never stop medications that are prescribed by a medical doctor without a medical consultation. You must taper off many medications. You cannot just stop medications suddenly without risking side effects. Your prescribing medical doctor should be involved in this process.

Acupuncturists do not prescribe pharmaceutical drugs. We often know the basics about your medications, but cannot give advice on pharmaceuticals.

In most cases, it is best to get acupuncture for a while before you try to stop medications of any sort. You want to treat the underlying problem before you quit medications. There can also be a rebound effect with some drugs. You could get symptoms that are worse than what you started with before you got a prescription. Your body has gotten used to having the drug and reacts when you stop taking it.

How much does acupuncture cost?

The cost varies, depending on your location and practitioner. The average is $60 to $85. The herbs usually cost extra, they range from $10 to $20 per bottle. Pharmaceutical grade herbs cost more than other brands. Each formula also has a different price; it depends on the herbs in the formula.

There are two types of acupuncture available. The first is "private" acupuncture. That is the most common way to get treatment in the West. You will have a private room for the consultation and treatment. You will be in the room alone for the duration of about 45 minutes to an hour.

The other type of acupuncture is "community acupuncture." Community acupuncture is done in a group setting. The cost ranges from $15 to $40 per treatment. It is usually done on a sliding scale. You pay what you can afford. It makes it possible for people of all incomes to get the care they need at a lower price.

Does insurance pay for acupuncture?

In order to understand the answer, you have to understand how insurance works. If you have private insurance, your employer negotiates a contract with the insurance company. Your employer tells the insurance company the types of treatments they want to pay for. They choose deductibles and determine how many sessions of different types of therapy, if any, they want to cover.

If your insurance does not "cover" acupuncture, it is because your company did not provide for that. Acupuncture is a very inexpensive form of treatment that can reduce medical costs by avoiding expensive medications and surgery.

Flexible spending accounts will usually cover acupuncture and often Chinese herbs. Remember, flexible spending accounts are your money, it is not insurance. You should be reimbursed for acupuncture and Chinese herbs. The Chinese herbs are prescribed and are medicine.

Do I have to believe in it for it to work?

Your belief in acupuncture has no bearing on its effectiveness. We use specific points that affect your body in specific ways. You cannot stop it from working. If you have any doubts on this, check out all the animal acupuncture being done these days.

When will I start to feel better?

You will usually feel a difference within the first few treatments. You will continue to improve until you are as well as you are going to get. Even after you recover from your original ailment, getting acupuncture will improve the functioning of your body. It relieves stress, improves sleep, and improves digestion. It works on a very basic level to improve health.

What about the placebo effect?

Placebos are typically things like sugar pills. If you take a pill that has no medicinal benefit and get better anyway, that is called a placebo effect. You cannot get acupuncture without getting a benefit from it. Even if "sham" acupuncture points are used.

There are over 400 points on the body, what are the odds that you will get acupuncture and not hit an acupuncture point or a meridian? Your body has the ability to heal from a very small amount of acupuncture. Just treating one acupuncture point can have a profound effect on your health.

What to expect on your first visit.

On your first visit you will tell us what your symptoms are, we will look at your tongue, and take your pulse. We can easily tell you what your Chinese medicine diagnosis is. After a few treatments, we can see how you are responding and give you an idea of how long you will need to get care.

What about all those images of people with needles in their faces?

I don't like it when they put 100 needles in someone's face or head for dramatic effect in movies or pictures. I rarely use points on the face, especially on new patients. When I do, it is to put a few needles in the forehead to relax wrinkles out, or to do Large Intestine 20 by the nose, to open the sinuses if a patient has sinus pain.

You can actually get what is called an "acupuncture facelift." Acupuncture is done on specific points on the face which act as trigger points to relax muscles. Wrinkles are caused by either saggy skin or tension in the facial muscles that causes lines. Acupuncture relaxes muscles; it is a good alternative to Botox. Botox freezes the muscles, acupuncture just relaxes them.

The lines between your eyes are easy to get rid of. It will take about four treatments in total to completely get rid of them. You will usually be able to tell a difference after one visit. You can also get acupuncture to treat other health issues when you get a face treatment. We treat the whole person. It is hard to look good when you are not getting enough sleep or are stressed out.

I always offer it as an option to get a few wrinkles ironed out in each session of acupuncture. It is very easy to reduce frown lines with acupuncture.

Will I bleed?

Occasionally you can bleed a tiny drop from certain points. If you have needles in your leg and you move your leg while lying down during your treatment, you might bleed a tiny amount, when the needles are removed. You will not gush blood, as some people expect.

If you have weak blood vessels, you are more likely to bleed. In fact, it is to your advantage to get acupuncture and find out if you bleed easily. It will tell you how strong your veins are. If you have weak veins in your legs, you will also have weak veins in other parts of your body.

The quality and health of your leg veins is the same as the ones in your heart. To strengthen veins, I recommend taking Tru OPCs by Nature's Way. This is grape seed extract. Other brands are not as good, so I recommend that one exclusively.

I've had patients refuse to spend any money on that, wanting to take something they already bought. They will continue to bleed when they get acupuncture, until they take the correct brand. That is why I know that Tru OPCs are the best.

How do you find the acupuncture points?

We find acupuncture points by what we call "bony landmarks." For example, we measure down from the knee by using our hands as a measurement. We also measure from the medial malleolus, which is the round bone on the inside of your ankle. This bone is used to locate points on the spleen meridian and kidney meridians.

Spleen 6 is a commonly used point. It is one hand-width above the medial malleolus, behind the calf bone. This point is one of the most commonly used on the body. It regulates hormones, improves sleep, relieves stress, improves digestion, and helps your body to get rid of excess fluid. The medial malleolus is the round bone one the inside of your ankle.

The quality of your sleep is always discussed when you get acupuncture. If you are not sleeping well, you will not heal well, so it is always a part of your treatment. In fact, it would be impossible not to treat your sleep. The acupuncture points that are used for other issues also improve the underlying cause of your insomnia.

Please be aware that each acupuncturist will have his/her choice of acupuncture points. If you get acupuncture in one office and decide to go to a different office, the new acupuncturist might not treat the same points you had at the first office. Even if you continue with the same acupuncturist, the points you have treated can *differ with each treatment.* You can make requests of points you would like to have treated, but if that acupuncturist does not feel it is appropriate for you, you should respect that.

There are many different ways to give acupuncture. There are Chinese, Japanese, and Korean to name a few. You also can have TCM points, the Dr. Tan points, and the Dr. Tong points. Your acupuncturist will have point preferences based on his/her experience and education. Each system is different. You can benefit from all of them.

Acupuncture can be done locally, on the site of the pain, or distally, on a point that is not close to the site of the pain. The point choice is made based on your diagnosis and what is appropriate for you at that time. Your points might change every time you get acupuncture.

The points I have described in this book are TCM points. They are very commonly used and well known. TCM stands for Traditional Chinese Medicine. Acupuncture is thousands of years old. It is a rich medicine with a lot of ways to achieve your goal of health.

Chapter 20

Chinese Herbal Medicine

When you get acupuncture, you will often be prescribed Chinese herbs to take. You can take herbal formulas such as *Gui pi wan* during the day, to treat the heart energy and other formulas such as *An shen bu shen* to take in the evening to calm you down.

When you take Chinese herbs, you can fully recover from your insomnia. There is no need to take them long term. In many cases, you can recover completely in less than 6 weeks. Of course, combining the acupuncture with the herbs is the fastest route to good sleep.

In China, some herbal remedies are sold over the counter. Just like you go to the store to buy aspirin, they go to the store to buy herbs for their ailments

A few popular insomnia remedies:

An mian pian- This is used in the evening and before bed to calm the heart.

One of my favorite formulas for sleep is *Restful Sleep* from Golden Flower Chinese Herbs. This formula is the strongest one I have found for yin deficiency type insomnia. I have patients take it in the evening only.

Your acupuncturist will be able to diagnose you and recommend the best sleep formula for your particular case. This brand is not sold over the counter.

I am not listing all the possible Chinese medicine diagnoses that might cause insomnia, because there are many and you need a professional and thorough diagnosis for best results. If you try to treat yourself with Chinese herbs, it can take a long time of trying different remedies to see which ones help you. Your exact diagnosis determines which herbal formula, of the hundreds of formulas sold, is right for you.

Chinese herbs come in a variety of formats:

Raw herbs – these are boiled and the tea is drunk as directed. This is the traditional way of taking herbs in China. Since Americans are not used to this, few practitioners practice this.

Tablets and capsules of herbal extracts – most formulas can be purchased in tablet form. There are several brands in the US that are "pharmaceutical grade." They are processed in factories in Taiwan, in the same factories as pharmaceuticals. This gives them the same high quality assurance as pharmaceuticals. Tests are done on the herbs before they are boiled in big vats, to ensure the correct herb and active ingredients.

Herbal powders- the formulas are pre-cooked and the dehydrated extract can be prescribed. The formula can be more specific to suit your needs. This powder is combined with hot water to make a tea.

Chinese patent medicine – these are herbs in pellet form, exported from China. These are the type that are sold over the counter. Some formulas are only sold by Chinese manufacturers. This type is called "Tea pills." A bottle of teapills contains about 200 small pellets.

Chinese herbs are taken 2-3 times per day. Each time you take the herbs, you are improving your health. Even if you are only able to take it once per day, you will get better. It is more effective to take it more often.

Gui Pi Tang – Ginseng and Longan

Gui Pi Tang is the name of this formula in Chinese. You can also call it Ginseng and Longan. This formula has been used for hundreds of years. It was developed in *1253 AD*. This formula is one of the most prescribed herbal formulas in Chinese medicine.

Common Indications for Ginseng and Longan:
- Heart palpitations (You feel your heart beating)
- Anxiety
- Worry
- Restlessness
- Inability to concentrate or remember things

- Insomnia at night with fatigue during the day

Ginseng and Longan strengthens the digestion and calms the heart energy. Emotional issues always have a physical cause in Chinese medicine. When you treat the underlying cause of the emotional imbalance, the physical problem is improved as well. There is absolutely no separation of the mental from the physical. In fact, every emotion has a corresponding organ. For example, if you have too much fear, it affects your kidneys. This weakens your kidneys over time and can cause symptoms such as frequent urination and low back pain.

If you do not have good digestion, you will not be healthy. That is why we always treat the digestion when you get acupuncture. With good digestion, you will have good energy and your body will be able to extract what it needs from the food you eat to heal from whatever ailment you have.

The ingredients for Ginseng and Longan are:
Panax Ginseng or Codonopsis – Ginseng is used to strongly boost energy and digestion. Codonopsis is used as a less expensive and gentler substitute for ginseng.

Longan – Improves blood in the heart and supports digestion. Calms the spirit (relieves stress and anxiety). Improves memory and treats dizziness from blood deficiency.

Astragalus – Strengthens digestion. It improves energy levels. It is also used to strengthen the immune system to improve resistance to colds and flu. Treats lack of appetite and fatigue.

Atractylodes- strengthens the digestion, helps reduce excess fluid retention (edema). It treats fatigue.
Poria – Improves digestion, reduces excess fluid retention. Calms the spirit.

Dang gui- Nourishes the blood. Regulates the menses and can help treat anemia or blood deficiency.
Zizyphus seed –Nourishes blood and calms the spirit. It is used as a sedative to treat the underlying cause of insomnia.

Senega root, Polygala – A very sedating herb that calms the spirit. Used for insomnia, palpitations, anxiety, and restlessness.

Licorice root – Used to improves digestion and energy levels. It is also used to stop coughing, relieve muscle spasms and harmonize herbal formulas.

I have only listed very basic descriptions of these herbs. I also have not included the Chinese names on purpose. I want this book to be a practical guide.

You will notice that half this formula improves digestion and energy levels and the other half treats the heart energy by sedating it. The heart has to have energy to be healthy. The combination of energy tonics and spirit calming herbs are what makes this formula so useful for so many things.

There are different variations of this formula. All herbal formulas can be modified with the addition of other herbs to make it useful for other things. It is most often used with the above formula.

If this formula is appropriate for you, your acupuncturist might also combine it with other herbs to treat other ailments. This formula is very strong to improve energy levels. It is also used for rejuvenation after a long period of illness. It is called "Spleen returning" to show how it helps recover the health by treating the digestion and heart energy.

Gui Pi Tang is the name of the powder. "Tang" means powder or decoction. "Wan" and "Pian" mean tablets.

Chapter 21

What is Your Chinese Medicine Diagnosis?

This is a short questionnaire that will help you understand how diagnosis is done in Chinese medicine. Note that these symptoms and diagnoses have nothing to do with what modern medicine would use. It is also very common to have multiple symptoms in each category. When you get that organ treated, all the symptoms in that category go away.

Acupuncture can treat most ailments at the same time. Each acupuncture point has multiple functions and affects several organs to treat the underlying cause of your health issue. *If you would like to print this out, it is on my website, www.acupunctureexplained.com.*

I like to use this long list of symptoms, because my patients forget how many problems they had when they first started getting acupuncture. I have them fill this form in when they first come to my office. They then fill out the form after 6 weeks of treatment. We compare the two versions. So many unusual symptoms that seem unrelated go away when you get acupuncture.

Overall Temperature-(Kidney function):

Cold hands
Cold fingers
Cold feet
Cold toes
Sweaty hands
Sweaty feet
Hot body temperature (sensation)
Cold body temperature (sensation)
Afternoon hot flashes
Night sweats
Heat in the hands, feet, and chest
Hot flashes any time of the day
Thirsty
Perspire easily
Lack of perspiration

Overall energy--(Lung, Kidney function):

Shortness of breath
Difficulty keeping eyes open in the daytime
General weakness
Easily catch colds
Fatigue
Feel worse after exercise

Blood:

Dizziness
See floating black spots

Heart Energy:

Palpitations
Anxiety
Sores on the tip of the tongue
Restlessness
Mental confusion
Frequent dreams
Wake unrefreshed

Lung function:

Nasal Discharge
Cough
Nose Bleeds
Sinus Congestion
Dry mouth
Dry throat
Dry Nose
Dry Skin
Allergies
Alternating fever and chills
Sneezing
Headache
Overall achy feeling in the body

135

Stiff shoulders
Sore throat
Difficulty breathing
Sadness

Spleen function:

Low appetite
Abrupt weight gain or loss
Abdominal bloating
Abdominal gas
Gurgling noise in the stomach
Fatigue after eating
Prolapsed organs
Easily bruised
Over-thinking
Worry

Spleen, Stomach, Large Intestine, Small Intestine function:

Loose stools
Constipated
Diarrhea
Undigested food in stools

Dampness trapped in the body:

General sensation of heaviness in the body
Mental heaviness
Mental sluggishness

Mental fogginess
Swollen hands or feet
Swollen joints
Chest congestion
Nausea
Snoring

Stomach function:

Burning sensation after eating
Large appetite
Bad breath
Bleeding, swollen, or painful gums
Acid reflux
Ulcer (diagnosed)
Belching
Hiccoughs
Stomach pain

Liver, Gall Bladder function:

Alternating diarrhea and constipation
Chest pain
Tight sensation in the chest
Bitter taste in the mouth
Anger easily
Frustration
Depression
Irritability
Skin rashes
Headache at the top of the head

Tingling sensation
Numbness
Muscle cramping
Grinding Teeth
Convulsions
Lump in the throat
Neck tension
Limited Range-of-Motion, Neck
Shoulder tension
High-pitched ringing in the ears

Kidney, Urinary Bladder function:

Sore knees
Weak knees
Low back pain
Memory problems
Excessive hair loss
Low-pitched ringing in the ears
Kidney stones
Bladder infections
Wake during the night twice or more to urinate
Lack of bladder control
Fear
Easily startled

For the printable version, my main website is www.acupunctureexplained.com.

Chapter 22

Other Sleep Issues

Teeth Grinding

If you grind your teeth at night, there are several possible causes of this. If you have a magnesium deficiency, your muscles can be too tight. Once the muscle becomes too tight, it will often stay that way. About 80% of us are deficient in magnesium. Magnesium is used by your body to relax muscles. If you do not have enough of it, you can easily develop tight muscles anywhere in your body.

Tight muscles can also lead to migraine headaches. The muscles in the neck and shoulders get tight over time and put pressure on the nerves that go to your head. When normal nerve function and blood flow are blocked, you have pain.

Once you develop teeth grinding, you will need to take supplemental magnesium for a while to build your blood levels back up. Your body will pull minerals from your bones when you do not have enough in your blood. The bones need to be replenished also.

Another possible cause of teeth grinding is stress. This is the diagnosis in Chinese medicine. Stress makes your body tight. Over time, the muscles get tighter and tighter and put pressure on the nerves. Acupuncture in the jaw area can relax the muscles that are causing you to clench your jaw. Once the muscles have been over-used and tight, taking magnesium alone might not be enough.

Please see the calcium/magnesium deficiency chapter in this book for more information.

Snoring and Sleep Apnea

Food allergies are a common cause of snoring. Dairy of any kind causes an increase in phlegm or mucus. Your body cannot digest dairy well because the enzymes you need to digest it are not made by humans.

When you eat dairy, your body cannot digest it well. Your body makes excess mucus to protect you from the irritation of undigested proteins. It also inflames the tissue to protect you.

Dairy is also a common cause of sinus and allergy symptoms. You can stop all dairy for a few days and see if you improve.

If you want to use milk, there are many options. My favorite one is coconut milk. I like *Coconut Dream.* Other popular types of non-dairy milk are rice milk and almond milk. Almond milk is available at most grocery stores.

Common symptoms of food allergies:

- Coughing while eating or 30 minutes to an hour afterwards. This is your body trying to defend itself from the food it finds offensive.
- Sneezing while or after eating. Your body is trying to get rid of the thing it is allergic to.
- Feeling a lump in your throat. This can be allergies or Hashimoto's Auto-immune Thyroiditis. Your immune system attacks the thyroid and it feels like you are being choked. You also can feel like you have something in your throat that you cannot swallow or cough up, it is just stuck there. If it is allergies or food sensitivities, your body will make mucus in your throat to protect you.

In Chinese medicine theory, snoring is caused by excess phlegm. The excess phlegm or mucus is caused by weak digestion. If you are not digesting your food well, you can have excess mucus. This can also cause allergy symptoms. There are herbal formulas to treat allergies, but if your digestion is weak, they might not be enough.

It is very easy to treat weak digestion with Chinese medicine. Acupuncture points can improve digestion and resolve excess phlegm. Herbs are also prescribed. One of the most popular remedies for digestion is called Six Gentlemen. Your acupuncturist can put you on the formula that is best for you.

Pinellia is the herb that is used to resolve phlegm/mucus. This is in an herbal formula called Six Gentlemen. A word of caution, I do not recommend self-treating for this. Panax ginseng is often in Six gentlemen and it can be contraindicated for people with high blood pressure. It is not a problem for everyone, but it is best to see an herbalist if you have high blood pressure. In the right herbal formula, ginseng could be appropriate for your health issue.

Panax ginseng is used in many herbal formulas and in several formulas that are used to rejuvenate the heart energy. It can revive your system and improve your energy levels when used correctly. It is not usually used alone as a single herb. It is used in small amounts and combined with other herbs. That makes it less likely to cause a problem.

Chapter 23

Leg cramps at night

If you have leg cramps, you can wake up in the middle of the night in agony. Often this is caused by a mineral deficiency. The most common deficiencies are: calcium, magnesium, and potassium. If you do not have enough minerals, your muscles will be tight.

There is also the chance that you have a diagnosis in Chinese medicine of a liver blood deficiency. That is similar to anemia, but it is a Chinese medicine syndrome. If you have a blood deficiency, your muscles do not have enough blood in them to function properly. The muscles get tight to try to restore normal blood flow.

Liver blood deficiency common symptoms are:

- Floaters (black spots floating in front of your eyes). Look at a white wall and see if you see black spots floating around. This is usually diagnosed as a liver blood deficiency. This can be treated.
- Insomnia

- Cramps
- Muscle spasms
- Weak muscles
- Blurred vision

You only need to have one symptom here that could indicate a liver blood deficiency. One formula that can be used for this is Xiao yao wan. This is also called Free and Easy Wanderer. It soothes and regulates your liver energy and improves blood levels.

Bupleurum Calmative Compound from Planetary Herbals is an over the counter remedy for your liver. This formula is so good for stress that I have often wished they would just put it in our water supply. Most people can benefit from this. You can see your acupuncturist for formulas that are more appropriate for you, but this formula is one of the most popular in Chinese medicine.

Here are the ingredients and a description of how they work:

Dong Quai Root- Nourishes blood, relieves spasms
Atractylodes Rhizome—improves digestion and energy levels
Chinese Peony Root- Nourishes blood, relieves spasms
Poria Sclerotium – Improves digestion, reduces excess fluid in body

Ginger Root Extract (4:1)- harmonizes (helps herbs work better together)

Licorice Root Extract (4:1)- Nourishes blood, relieves spasms

Bupleurum Root Extract – Strongly regulates liver energy and relieves stress

Chinese Mint Extract (5:1)- cooling and relieves stress

Since 80% of us are deficient in magnesium, it can't hurt to take some to be sure this is not a cause of leg cramps or other health issues. A good quality calcium/magnesium product is *Raw Calcium* by Garden of Life. It is organic, so it is absorbed much better than other mineral supplements.

There is also a homeopathic remedy for leg cramps at night that might help. **Hylands Leg Cramps PM**.

Chapter 24

Staying Asleep

There is a difference in sleeping problems between getting to sleep and staying asleep. When you are under 40, it is more common to have problems getting to sleep. That is often correlated with the heart energy.

After the age of 40, you suffer a decline in hormones and a problem staying asleep can occur. This is called a kidney yin deficiency.

You might have heard of yin and yang and wondered what they were. Yin and yang are the foundation of life. To make things simple, I will explain how these principles are used in Chinese herbs.

Yin is cool and moist and yang is hot and dry. As you get older, you have a decline in both yin and yang. You can see these as hormones. Your body does not make enough hormones as you get older. It is a natural decline of aging. The good news is that you can treat this decline with acupuncture and herbs.

Some common symptoms of a kidney yin deficiency are:

- Hot flashes
- Dry eyes
- Vaginal dryness
- Irritability

A yin deficiency can be correlated with a decline in estrogen and progesterone. Your body is just not making the same amount of hormones as you were younger. If you can treat this, you can improve your quality of life as you get older. You can take herbal tonics long term to fight the signs of aging. Or, you can just take them until your symptoms go away. In China, herbal tonics are very popular and are used regularly to reduce the symptoms of aging.

A yang deficiency can be correlated with a decline in testosterone. This deficiency can be treated easily with Chinese medicine. It usually takes less than a month.

Some common symptoms of a kidney yang deficiency are:

- Low back pain
- Frequent urination
- Waking at night to urinate
- Incontinence – including sneezing incontinence
- Low libido

Just because it is normal to have a decline in hormones as you age, does not mean you cannot treat it and improve your overall health as a result.

For a kidney yin deficiency, you can take American ginseng. American ginseng is considered a supreme tonic and is highly valued in China. Most of our American ginseng is grown in Wisconsin.

If you have a problem staying asleep, it will take longer to treat than the problem of getting to sleep. To restore your kidney yin will take several months. It is as simple as taking daily herbs.

A good kidney tonic is Cordyceps Sinensis. This herb will strengthen your kidney yin and yang. It will boost the energy of your kidneys, lungs, and heart. Planetary Herbals makes a good cordyceps product, it is called Cordyceps 450. I also like the cordyceps from Nature's Way. Most people feel improved energy levels within a week of starting this. It is a good tonic for men and women.

The best quality American ginseng I have found is American ginseng extract from Sun Ten Herbs. It is available over the counter. One capsule is all that is necessary if you take a top quality extract.

Chapter 25

Acupuncture Points for Insomnia

Acupuncture improves energy levels, balances hormones and regulates the body. Your body knows what healthy is, you just need to help it by improving energy levels and regulating circulation so it can restore healthy function.

Most people need to improve energy levels and recover from stress. These are the most common ailments we treat, in addition to pain.

Here are a few acupuncture points and a description of how they work.

Stomach 36

Stomach 36 is used to improve digestion, and improve energy levels. This is one of the most commonly used acupuncture points. It also regulates your stomach and intestines. Most diseases include fatigue and digestive weakness. You will recover faster from your illness if you can digest your food and have better energy levels. This point will help *any ailment* related to your stomach or intestines, including acid reflux. It regulates the energy of these organs and helps restore normal function.

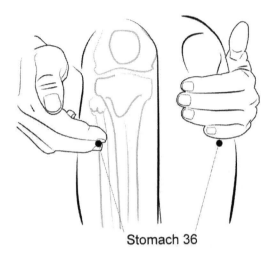

Stomach 36

The easiest way to locate Stomach 36 is by placing the hand over the eye of the knee. The point is located just below the hand.

Heart 7

Heart 7 is used to calm the heart, resolve insomnia and anxiety.

Heart 7 is located on the wrist crease, on the thumb side of the ulnaris tendon. Pressing on this point can be very effective to relieve anxiety and insomnia.

Heart 5 in this image is used to regulate the heart energy, and resolve palpitations. It is used to regulate heart rhythm.

Pericardium 6

Pericardium 6 calms the heart, regulates your stomach (helpful for nausea and morning sickness). Acupressure can be used on this point. See the chapter on acupressure for more details. This is one of the most effective points for insomnia. It relieves stress, anxiety, and is very relaxing.

Pericardium 6 and Heart 7 are the most important acupressure points for insomnia. They also relieve anxiety.

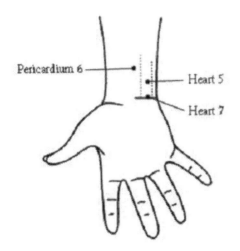

Pericardium 6 — •

Heart 5

Heart 7

Liver 3

Liver 3 is the most important point for stress. It regulates your liver energy, which is how Chinese medicine diagnoses stress. Stress affects your liver energy, when your liver energy is out of balance, it can cause:

- Migraines
- Increased sensitivity to stress
- PMS
- Fatigue
- Digestive disorders
- Infertility
- Insomnia

Any disease that is worse when you are under stress is probably caused by a liver energy imbalance. It will be improved by using this point.

Doing acupressure on this point can be very effective to relieve stress. I suggest using a mini massager. You can do this point on both feet.

Liver 3 is located by putting your index finger on the area between your big toe and second toe. You will feel a dip in the fleshy area between your toes. Acupressure in this location will cover a large enough area, you should not be concerned you will miss the point.

Liver

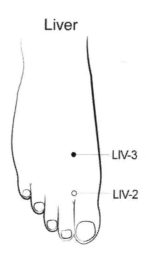

155

Liver 2 is used for what we call "Liver fire", this is an extreme reaction to stress. You will need an acupuncturist to help you with this. Liver fire entails more "heat", you will tend to get a flushed face when you lose your temper. That is only one symptom of this pattern.

Spleen 6

Spleen 6 is a major point on that body that does dozens of things. It regulates hormones, strengthens kidneys and spleen, regulates liver energy (treats stress), Tonifies blood (similar to anemia). This point is very calming and can be used in the evening to relax. I use this point on most patients. It also helps get rid of excess fluid in the body (edema).

It is located by placing your hand on the medial malleolus bone, which is the bony protuberance on the inside of your ankle. This point is located behind the leg bone. Each person needs to have his/her hand used as the measurement. For example, if you are treating someone smaller than you, you will need to adjust the measurement size.

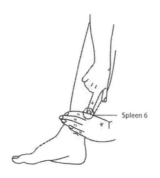
Spleen 6

Kidney Deficiency

Another imbalance that often causes insomnia is a kidney weakness. The kidney energy gets weaker as you get older, in Chinese medicine theory. You can easily improve the energy of your kidneys by getting acupuncture and taking Chinese herbs. This will improve longevity and treat problems such as back pain, fatigue, and hormone problems.

A kidney deficiency correlates to a hormone deficiency. Your body is not making enough hormones to function in a healthy way. The most common symptoms of a kidney deficiency are: Low back pain, knee pain, frequent urination, incontinence, fatigue, insomnia, and nighttime urination.

One of the most relaxing points to use on the kidney meridian is Kidney 6.

Kidney 6

Kidney 6 is used to relieve hot flashes, calm the heart, improve hormones via strengthening the kidneys, and improve overall energy levels. This point is below the medial malleolus, which is, the ball on the inside of the ankle. This point is so relaxing that I sometimes do not use it on patients who have to go back to work after their acupuncture treatment.

The heart and kidneys are the most common organs that affect your ability to sleep. Another issue with sleep is when you wake up during the night. This is covered in detail in the chapter "Are your kidneys waking you up?"

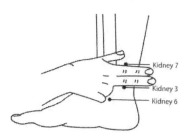

Some of the most common diagnoses that cause insomnia are:

Heart Qi and Blood deficiency - this is caused by long term stress and anxiety weakening your digestion, which weakens the heart energy. What we call heart energy has no correlation to Western medicine. You will not find this problem on a test from your medical doctor. It is a diagnosis that has been used for thousands of years to treat illnesses.

A few possible symptoms of heart qi and blood deficiency are:

- Palpitations – when you feel your heart beating. This often happens when you lie in bed at night and cannot fall asleep.

- Fatigue - your digestion is not good and your energy levels are low, so you will not have good energy.
- Easily startled
- Anxiety
- Insomnia
- Poor memory.

You do not need to have all these symptoms to have a diagnosis of heart qi and blood deficiency. This is a very common diagnosis.

Acupuncture points that can be used to treat this include: Stomach 36, Spleen 6, and Pericardium 6.

Acupuncture should be received once per week, twice if you can. The more often you get treatments, the faster you get better. Every time you get acupuncture, the organs that are involved with your insomnia and other health issues are regulated and strengthened. You will often recover from symptoms that you did not even realize you had. If you cannot get acupuncture weekly, just discuss it with your acupuncturist. We are used to working within people's budgets to help them. Do not hesitate to discuss this.

The most important thing is that you stick with the program until you get better. If you can see an acupuncturist for an herbal consultation every few weeks, that is also an affordable option. The herbs heal you just like the acupuncture.

To find a good acupuncturist, look for someone who has a license. Most states license acupuncturists and require a 3 year Graduate degree in order to qualify. There are also several national board exams that have to be passed to be licensed.

If your acupuncturist is licensed, the initials are L.Ac.. That stands for Licensed Acupuncturist. Each state in the US has different titles. In Rhode Island, it is Doctor of Acupuncture. In New Mexico, it is a Doctor of Oriental Medicine, DOM. You can just ask if the person attended graduate school and if she was licensed by the state.

Other types of practitioners are allowed to practice acupuncture with a small amount of training. Each state has different required levels of training. In some states, there is no special training necessary for someone who is already a medical practitioner, to be "certified" to do acupuncture. Since a licensed acupuncturist is in school for three to four years studying at a graduate level, you should get better and faster results with him/her.

Chinese herbal medicine

Chinese herbs are medicine. You take the herbal formula to address the underlying imbalances causing your symptoms. You can combine herbs with acupuncture for a faster effect, or take Chinese herbs alone if you prefer. You can go to an acupuncturist and get a prescription for herbs. Please be patient with the healing process. It takes time to recover. You are treating the root of the problem, so once you get better, you stay well.

You will notice fast results with acupuncture, but you will need to continue with your care for a complete healing. Most people need at least 4 sessions, or a month, to recover. It also depends on your diagnosis; some diseases take longer than others.

The more problems you have, the longer it takes to get better. We can treat many of your ailments at the same time, but your body does the healing. Your overall health will determine how long that takes.

Your acupuncturist will work with you on your treatment schedule. Ideally you would get acupuncture twice per week, but even every other week is better than not at all. Just do not give up.

Chapter 26

Your Best Night's Sleep

This is a summary of what you need to do to recover from chronic insomnia.

Vitamins and Herbs

Take your vitamins to ensure you are getting everything you need to be healthy. Take Garden of Life Vitamin Code *Raw Multi vitamins, Raw Calcium*, and *vitamin C*.

You treat your adrenal fatigue with licorice root and Siberian ginseng as well as high doses of vitamin C. Take herbal tonics to improve digestion and energy levels throughout the day.

Get Acupuncture on Your Lunch Hour

Acupuncture points:

Spleen 6- Is used to balance hormones, strengthen your kidneys and spleen and regulate your liver to relieve stress.

Liver 3- Is used to relieve stress and regulate your hormones via your liver energy.

Stomach 36 – Is used to strengthen digestion, improve energy levels, strengthen immune system and regulate your elimination.

Kidney 3, 6, and 7 –Is used to strengthen your kidneys. It also improves hormone levels, reduces nighttime urination, and reduces hot flashes. These points are especially good for insomnia.

Evening Supplements

Calcium and Magnesium – relax your muscles, improve sleep.

Take your evening herbs, either prescribed Chinese herbal medicine or over the counter Valerian root formula. Take these herbs at least 2 hours before bedtime. It is best to give them time to start working.

Two hours before bed, you can do acupressure on Pericardium 6 and Heart 7. This will start to calm you and help you stay asleep.

In bed, use your Bach Rescue Sleep. Spray a few times in your mouth. You can repeat as needed. If you wake at night, you can use more flower essences to get back to sleep.

Your essential oils like lavender can be rubbed on your wrists or misted on your pillow.

You can use your white noise CD or machine if needed to block out external noise.

Updates to This Book

As I find new supplements, I will list them on my main website, www.AcupunctureExplained.com. I will also provide links to some products.

I have done extensive research on the available over-the-counter supplements for sleep. I excluded supplements with synthetic melatonin. I do research all the time and when I find something new, that I can recommend, I will put it on my site.

Resources

The Illustrated Encyclopedia of Healing Remedies by C. Norman Shealy – If you want to get one book on natural remedies, get this one. It includes Chinese herbs, Western herbs, Ayurveda, flower essences, homeopathy, and aromatherapy.

Natural Health Encyclopedia of Herbal Medicine – DK by Andrew Chevallier. Well illustrated with 550 herbs. It also includes Chinese names of herbs. This is a good reference to help in the study of Chinese herbal remedies.

Herbal Remedies, Eyewitness Companion--DK by Andrew Chevallier. This is a smaller book, with 140 herbs. It is well illustrated. If you want to buy one book on herbs, this is the one to get.

Backyard Medicine- by Julie Bruton-Seal and Matthew Seal

Little Herb Encyclopedia by Jack Ritchason N.D.

Acupuncture and Chinese Medicine Books:

Between Heaven and Earth by Harriet Beinfield and Efrem Korngold. I used this book extensively in my first year in acupuncture school. It explains Chinese medicine very thoroughly.

The Ancient Wisdom of Chinese Tonic Herbs by Ron Teeguarden. How Chinese tonic herbs can improve energy and vitality.

A Manual of Acupuncture by Peter Deadman, Mazin Al-Khafaji and Kevin Baker. This is the acupuncture point location and indication book that acupuncture students use to learn the points. It has an excellent index in the back that will help you learn what each acupuncture point does and how to locate it.

The Foundations of Chinese Medicine by Giovanni Maciocia. This is the first year text for acupuncture students. It explains Chinese medicine diagnosis and Chinese medicine theory.

The Practice of Chinese Medicine by Giovanni Maciocia. This is the second year book for acupuncture students. Dozens of diseases are explained in Chinese medicine terms. It explains how you diagnose different diseases, which acupuncture points to use and which herbal formulas to use.

167

The Way of Herbs by Michael Tierra

The Way of Chinese Herbs by Michael Tierra. This is a great reference for single Chinese herbs and Chinese herbal medicine formulas.

Chinese Herbal Medicine, Formulas and Strategies by Dan Bensky. This book explains hundreds of herbal formulas and how they work. It is used by third year acupuncture students.

Chinese Herbal Medicine, Materia Medica by Dan Bensky. This has hundreds of single Chinese herbs. Their temperature, meridians, organs and functions are explained. This is a second year acupuncture student book.

Recommended flower essence books:

Bach Flower Therapy, Theory and Practice by Mechthild Scheffer. If you get one book, get this one.

The Encyclopedia of Bach Flower Therapy by Mechthild Scheffer.

The New Encyclopedia of Flower Remedies by Clare G. Harvey. This book includes flower essences from all over the world.

Handbook of Bach Flower Remedies for Animals by Enric Homedes. This book includes how to treat shelter animals and animals that have been abandoned.

Bach Flower Remedies for Animals by Helen Graham and Gregory Vlamis.

The Flower Remedy Book by Jeffrey Garson Shapiro. This book has 700 flower essences categorized by emotional issues.

Flower Essence Repertory – by Patricia Kaminski. This is the main book that explains FES flower essences in detail. It includes Bach flower essences.

About the Author

Deborah Bleecker, L.Ac., M.S.O.M. has a Master of Science degree in Oriental Medicine.

In 1995 she developed a repetitive stress injury on the job. Her problems included nerve pain and chronic inflammation. She saw many medical doctors, but received no relief. She was told that there was no cure for nerve pain. She was also not responding to their treatment for inflammation. There was nothing they could offer. She was told to get used to the pain, as it would be permanent.

She was not interested in accepting a pronouncement that she would have chronic pain the rest of her life, so she started doing research on natural remedies. She determined that acupuncture seemed to be a cure for everything and gave it a try. She started feeling better and knew that with time and perseverance she would completely recover. In fact, she was cured of the "incurable" nerve pain.

She graduated from acupuncture school in 1999 and has been studying Chinese medicine and other natural remedies since then.

Printed in Great Britain
by Amazon